THERAPEUTIC HYPNOSIS

THERAPEUTIC HYPNOSIS

Michael M. Miller, M.D.

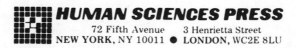 **HUMAN SCIENCES PRESS**
72 Fifth Avenue   3 Henrietta Street
NEW YORK, NY 10011 ● LONDON, WC2E 8LU

ISBN: 0-87705-341-3

Copyright © 1979 by Human Sciences Press
72 Fifth Avenue, New York, New York 10011

Printed in the United States of America
9 987654321

Library of Congress Cataloging in Publication Data

Miller, Michael M.
  Therapeutic hypnosis

  Includes bibliographical references and index.
  1. Hypnotism—Therapeutic use. I. Title.
RC495.M52   615'.8512   78-10405
ISBN 0-87705-341-3

CONTENTS

CONTENTS

PREFACE

The art of therapeutic hypnosis has had a painful birth. After Anton Mesmer was discredited by medical authority in Vienna and Paris, and then dealt a crowning blow by the French Academy, the practice and development of clinical hypnosis was set back for almost a century. Freud's rejection of hypnosis and his promotion of psychoanalysis further retarded the development of hypnosis as a healing art. It is evident that had Freud not gone to study hypnosis with Janet, Charcot and Bernheim, the theory of psychoanalysis would not have evolved.

The literature on hypnosis is extensive and there are a number of texts which deal primarily with introductory concepts and methods. While the current work will be of interest to students in the field, it will have particular utility for those who are already practicing hypnotherapy.

I have felt that most books on clinical hypnosis, with the exception of a few, have dealt more with theory than with clinical practice. I have sought in this work to present my own observations, conclusions and practices that in the course of my extensive use of hypnotherapy over the past 25 years have proven to be of pragmatic clinical value. Therefore, I am presenting here procedures which I have found to be highly effective and time-saving as well.

I have included a chapter dealing with my original work in hypnoaversion therapy which has already proven of great value to large numbers of patients suffering from chronic alcoholism, nicotinism, obesity and other conditions. Furthermore, in utilizing hypnoaversion in conjunction with psychotherapy I have successfully treated homosexuals of the bisexual type and have found this procedure to hold promise as an adjunctive in the treatment of selected cases of incipient, overt homosexuality.

I have not attempted to cover the extensive literature on hypnosis nor all of the varied hypnotic techniques. For the sake of brevity and practicality, I have limited myself primarily to those concepts and procedures which have proven of genuine value in practice.

Chapter 1

HISTORICAL BACKGROUND OF HYPNOTHERAPY

Hypnotherapy, in the form of both waking and sleep suggestion, is among the oldest of the healing arts and has been practiced since ancient times. In Asia, Persian magi and Hindu fakirs awed their subjects with their abilities to intensify cataleptic states by maintaining strong fixation of the eyes on their subjects. The Hindu temple priest and his Yogi and Fakir brothers impressed believers with their fatiguing, repetitive rituals, monotonous chants and prayers. Such feats and practices supported their claims of possessing supernatural powers of healing and influencing human behavior.

Primitive religion and witchcraft made use of the hypnotic method in ancient times, for example, in the so-called Egyptian "Temple Sleep" during which state curative utterances were suggested to sufferers by priests who employed hypnotic incense and chanting to further the induction of such states. The Abatons of the Greek Golden Age had "Sleep Temples of the Sick," where people were treated by prolonged sleep induced by repetitious rhetoric, soft music and drugs.

Trance states were induced by means of waking suggestion practiced by tribal witch doctors, magicians, medicine men and shamans, who employed drums, flutes, whirring and flashing fetish-like objects, head dresses and other adornments as well as ritual dances.

Similarly, techniques of waking suggestion (some subtle—some not so subtle) have been used to influence men since the beginning of history. For centuries such practices were held in high esteem and were sanctioned by the ruling powers, since they presented an often powerful instrument for influencing and controlling the ignorant and superstitious masses. Religious and magical healers often were able to greatly impress and influence backward peoples by means of magical and religious rites, sacrifices, pilgrimages, dress and religious ecstasies fanned by sacred ceremonies and rites. Suggestive influences were universally practiced among primitive peoples, ranging from simple symbolic fetishism and idol worship which protected against the evil spirits and forces—such as fire, flood, lightning and thunder—to more highly organized forms of worship with consolidation of power and authority in a single God (Monotheism). The practice of elaborate rituals, i.e., prayers, chanting, incense and impressive regal robes became widespread. Primarily waking suggestion, as exemplified by immersion in the Ganges of hordes of Hindu pilgrims, or faith healing as conducted at religious shrines such as Lourdes, again used the deep faith of the believer reinforced by examples of a miraculous recovery, i.e., a hysterical paralytic suddenly enabled to walk, etc. For man has always sought a magical solution to his problems.

The curative method was, for the most part, direct waking suggestion to alleviate symptoms of acute distress. On the whole, the church and the clergy, following in the footsteps of the earlier tribal magicians, medicine men and

witch doctors, recognized and exploited healing by faith
and suggestion. In fact, the medieval Christian Church on
the whole, made even more extensive use of symbolic, suggestive rituals and rites than did other religions. By means
of imposing architecture, often magnificent artistic works,
selective lighting and staging effects, darkening of the
church and illumination of the altar, incense, music, repetitious monotonous chanting enhanced by often remarkable
acoustics, sermons and prayer rituals, the individual was for
the most part overawed. As with hypnotic induction, the
individual was extolled to surrender with faith and devotion—to render himself unto God, meanwhile discarding,
at least for the time being, his critical reason and realistic
logic. It might be conjectured that only a Voltaire would
have been capable of withstanding it all without succumb-
ing. After a long process of conditioning and exposure to
religious rituals and rites, many individuals could no doubt
virtually enter into a hypnotic trance instantly upon smelling the incense. I had occasion to repeat this latter phenomena at my clinic experimentally. Here, we note the
phenomena of "dressage," in which the individual
becomes increasingly sensitized and responsive to hypnotic
suggestion so that the conditioned response becomes virtually instantaneous.

Thus, *waking* as well as *hypnotic* suggestion has been
effectively employed in various forms by the church for
centuries. The burdened and suffering, in their search for
peace of mind, security, love, absolution and immortality,
render themselves unto a loving father image anticipating
magical benefits and miracles and the lifting of their painful
burdens and responsibilities. Ironically, in spite of the wide
use of suggestion by the clergy, hypnosis as a healing art
was regarded as sacriligious in the western Christian world
all through the middle ages. In fact, even today, those
methods of psychotherapy which, of necessity, involved
psychic examination, analysis, intimate disclosures and

psychic influence, still meet with stern disapproval by some members of the clergy. The prerogative of the holy confessional was jealously safeguarded by the church for centuries. Because of the possibility of ecclesiastical reprisal the practice of hypnotherapy was often only carried on secretly, being regarded and banned by most religionists as witchcraft and the work of the devil. The healing influences of waking suggestion were likewise regarded with jealousy and as impinging on sacred religious practices and rites. Their use was not only declared sinful, but forbidden to the laity. Even the implementation of these methods by the healing professions was strongly discouraged and frowned upon. In medieval times, such healers might even have been roasted at the stake as heretics. Because of such strong opposition from the church primarily, hypnotic suggestion as a healing art fell into ill repute and literature concerning such practices was virtually unavailable.

MESMER

The revival of the ancient healing art of hypnotic suggestion was heralded into modern medical history during the eighteenth century by Franz Anton Mesmer, an Austrian physician. Mesmer (1734–1815) who deserves to be regarded as the father of medical hypnosis, was born at Iznang on Lake Constance. In his early years he had already revealed a high degree of imagination and versatility. He had broad interests and as a student pursued studies of philosophy, law and theology prior to obtaining his medical degree. He also revealed marked interest in astrology and music. In 1774 he became interested in magnetism as the result of the influence of a Jesuit, Father Maximilian Heil. It was at a time when significant new discoveries were being made in electrochemistry, electricity, magnetism and astronomy, and Mesmer was quick to explore the possible

therapeutic value of these new chemical and physical discoveries. As a result of the strong religious beliefs at the
time in faith and magical healing, he became preoccupied
with the "wonder cure" possibilities of magnetism. He
linked astrology and magnetism and began to relate health
to the concept that the individual must maintain a certain
electrochemical relationship with the heavenly bodies. Apparently, Mesmer was so interested in astrology that he
even completed a thesis in 1776 for his doctorate, "De
Planetarum Influxu" ("Concerning the Influence of the
Planets").

Soon after this, Mesmer began the practice of medicine in Vienna. He was able, because of an authoritative,
imaginative and persuasive personality to pursue a very
active social and professional life. Highly ambitious, he
began to court the wealthy widow of a former high ranking
officer of the Austrian Imperial Army, Anna Von Bosch,
whom he married. As a result, he was rapidly accepted
among the wealthy and aristocratic class.

His command of such new—and to the layman—overwhelming and mystical magical forces, gave him great influence, prestige, and power over his patients. Often a "pass"
or laying on of the hand was sufficient to induce a hypnotic
trance, although Mesmer was apparently unaware of the
psychic suggestive influence on his patients. Mesmer and
his patients believed that his "universal fluids" influenced
by the planets were largely responsible for these strange
effects.

As a result of his innovations and startling cures by
means of animal magnetism, he soon developed a very
large practice. However, as his practice grew and his amazing cures were publicized, there was considerable reaction
of envy and resentment among his professional colleagues.
Because Mesmer's results were not explainable in logical,
scientific terms, his work was regarded with scepticism and
he was rejected by the medical faculty of the University of

Vienna. Nevertheless, his fame spread throughout Europe and even attracted the attention of the Empress Maria Theresa. The Empress was very much interested in a child prodigy pianist whom she had made a protegé of hers, Maria Theresa Paradis. The child had suddenly become blind at the age of eight and Mesmer undertook to cure her of this disability. Since it was a case of hysterical blindness, he was able to restore her sight. However, the case was quite involved in that his patient, Maria, was the child of a very disturbed neurotic family. There was great tension in the family, apparently because of her parents' fear that Maria's restored vision would terminate the royal pension from the Empress. Because of this emotional upheaval in the family, Maria again developed blindness and the parents refused to continue her under Mesmer's care. This incident put Mesmer in disfavor with the Empress and certain of the officialdom and permitted his professional enemies to denounce and discredit him as a fraud.

As a result, in 1778, Mesmer decided to leave Vienna and to establish practice in Paris where he had certain contacts. Mesmer was able to get a Dr. Charles d'Eslon interested in his healing methods. Dr. d'Eslon was physician to the King's younger brother, the Comte d'Artois. D'Eslon became so interested that he joined with Mesmer in setting up a clinic. They were eminently successful and animal magnetism for a time became a "panacea." Mesmer soon had so many patients that he could not treat them individually, and so he contrived his famous so-called "baquets." These were large tubs filled with water. In them were bottles and iron filings. Attached to the bottles were numerous iron rods with handles which the patients were instructed to grasp so that the healing effects of the electrolytic fluids in the tubs could be transmitted to them. As they perceived these magnetic electrolytic effects, Mesmer walked among them and extolled their curative powers. With keen insight, he here cleverly and unknowingly utilized the potentiating suggestive influences of one subject upon another as they excitedly and emotionally conversed about the amazing effects they were experiencing. Their conversations set the scene for the first group hypnotherapy on record. Mesmer's subjects often regarded him with such awe and admiration that generally they were already highly susceptible and awaited the "great master physician" with grandiose expectation and marked anticipatory excitement.

This new art of healing was called "Mesmerism" after its discoverer. Mesmer's amazing feats in accomplishing sudden cures aroused a great deal of interest among certain of the younger and highly imaginative intellectual set, among whom the most notable was the Marquis de Puysegur, who was the first to describe the sleep-walking (somnambulistic) trance.

But again Mesmer's feats caused jealousy and enmity among the medical profession of his day. When, in certain instances, he failed to achieve a magical cure, they were quick to pounce upon him and publicly denounce his as a charlatan and a quack. In fact, Mesmer ultimately aroused such a storm of opposition that in 1784 his enemies succeeded in influencing King Louis XVI to set up a Royal Commission to investigate his practices. On the commission were such renowned scientists as Lavoisier, the chemist, our own Benjamin Franklin, the discoverer of the lightning rod who was also a member of the French Academy at that time, Bailly, the astronomer, Jussieu, the botanist, and Dr. Guillotin, soon to be known throughout the world as the creator of that instrument of death which struck such terror in the French Revolution. All of the members of the Commission were men highly recognized for their scientific gifts and judgment. That such an outstanding group of scientists were selected to sit in judgment of Mesmer is in itself a testimonial to the important status he had at that time. The Commission was determined to find out if the so-called "animal magnetism" existed and if it were beneficial or harmful to patients. They accordingly submitted themselves to the test of his methods and influence but were unable to perceive any actual effects upon themselves, therefore concluding that there was no genuine scientific foundation for the Mesmeric phenomena. They were of the opinion that the reported effects were a result of the overwhelming stimulation of the patient's imagination and that much harm could be done through the misuse of such unscientific methods. The Commission pointed out further that as a result of treatment several of Mesmer's patients had even developed new symptoms. The Commission condemned Mesmer as a quack without even offering him an opportunity to personally demonstrate the healing value of his methods.

It was unfortunate for Mesmer and mankind that this eminent Commission failed to comprehend the actual psychotherapeutic mechanisms involved. There is reason to conclude that the members may have broadened their investigation, but were undoubtedly influenced by the prevailing strong professional and scientific bias against Mesmer. They therefore sought out any facts with which they could indict him while failing utterly in reporting the positive results Mesmer had achieved with numerous patients. As a result, he lost his license to practice and was forced to retire, a broken and frustrated man, to a suburban life in Versailles. He then left France just before the outbreak of the French Revolution and retired in obscurity to Frauenfeld in Switzerland on the shores of his native Lake Constance. There, according to the most reliable information available, he lived a simple life, dedicating himself for the most part to treating poor patients of the area. This was an interesting turn from his heyday when he primarily treated the wealthy and aristocratic. When, in his declining years, Mesmer received an invitation to demonstrate his methods before the Prussian Academy in Berlin, he was apparently so embittered that he refused. He died three years later at Meersburg on March 5, 1815. Franz Anton Mesmer died but his art of healing through suggestion did not. No doubt, he died without ever really comprehending the mechanisms of suggestion which he had practiced so well and without realizing that he had set in motion a new orientation in medical psychology, which as Zilboorg pointed out, ultimately led to the deepest insights yet attained by man into the inner workings of the human mind.

ELLIOTSON AND BRAID

Mesmerism had been so thoroughly discredited in the report of the French Royal Commission that it was almost seventy years later before Elliotson and then Braid made an attempt to reevaluate and explore the medical therapeutic and scientific value of Mesmerism. Dr. John Elliotson, the founder of University College Hospital, London, was a highly creative medical scientist and one of the key figures in the history of English medicine. It was he who first introduced Laennec's stethoscope to England and who developed clinical procedures for examination of the heart and lungs which are standard even to this day. Elliotson began to experiment and practice with Mesmer's methods and as a result aroused considerable professional antagonism, particularly in orthodox medical circles. Elliotson had accepted Mesmer's theory of "animal magnetism" and made the error of defending it. In 1838, Thomas Wakely, the first editor and founder of the *Lancet*, tested Elliotson's claims that certain metals were more curative because they radiated more of this magnetic force. He then demonstrated that Elliotson was in error and that there was no difference in the effects produced on patients regardless of whether lead or nickel were employed. As a result, Elliotson was all too quickly labelled a fraud and not permitted to practice Mesmerism at the University Hospital. He immediately resigned his position as chief staff physician and professor at the medical school. In spite of this setback, Elliotson pursued his interest and was able, largely because of his splendid professional and scientific reputation and his strong personal influence, to interest others in Mesmerism and to stimulate further clinical research in this area. He established a Mesmeric hospital in London (Fitzroy Square), and in 1843 began publication of a journal called *Zoist* which was primarily devoted to Mesmerism and cranial physiology. It was due largely also to his personal influence that a number of Mesmeric hospitals were set up in London, Edinburgh, Dublin and several other large cities.

It was at about this time that James Braid, a Scotchman and Manchester surgeon, began to explore the medical and scientific value of Mesmerism, after he had witnessed a demonstration by LaFontaine, a relative of the great French writer of fables. It was in the pre-chloroform era and methods of anaesthesia were Braid's primary concern. Braid was so successful and enthusiastic about his initial experience in the clinical application of hypnotic suggestion that he sought to disseminate this technique among the medical profession at large. He was highly original in his approach to hypnosis, conducted research and developed the optic fixation induction procedure which to this day bears his name. Although the British Medical Association refused Braid's offer to demonstrate his method and to present a paper on the subject, he nevertheless remained undiscouraged, convinced of the importance of his work and carried on.

It was Braid who first used the term "hypnotism" and discussed the phenomena with which it dealt in a book entitled *Neurohypnology, or The Rationale of Nervous Sleep,* 1843 (New Rev. Ed. 1879, London: George Redway). At this time, Braid believed hypnosis to be based on a neurophysical phenomenon. It was not until years later, as a result of the extensive investigations of Liebeault and Bernheim, that he altered his opinion and accepted the thesis that the hypnotic sleep was in fact due to psychological factors. Since the "Braid" method was based on visual optic fixation, he was later very much impressed when he discovered that the blind could be hypnotized by verbal suggestion alone.

ESDAILE

Dr. James Esdaile, a young Scottish surgeon in India, after reading the initial reports of Elliotson and Braid, became quite interested and began to experiment with Mesmerism. Primarily because of the lack of a satisfactory means of anesthesia, he employed hypnosis and was reported to have performed over three hundred major and several thousand minor operations quite painlessly on patients under its influence, as well as to have reduced the mortality rate markedly. In spite of the accomplishments he claimed, the British medical journals refused to permit him to report his findings. However, he corresponded with Elliotson, reporting his results to him. Elliotson was most encouraging and publicized Esdaile's work in his journal, *Zoist.*

AMBROISE-AUGUST LIEBEAULT

Soon afterwards in France, about 1846, Dr. Ambroise-August Liebeault, a country physician, began to test Braid's methods. He discovered that by skillfully combining verbal sleep suggestion in conjunction with Braid's method of fixed gazing, that he was more effectively able to hypnotize patients. He perfected this technique to the point where he was able to induce trances in 85% of his patients. Liebeault's modification of Braid's method has become standard technique to this day. Some twenty years after his initial research, Dr. Liebeault wrote a book entitled, *Du Sommeil* (1866). At the time of its publication hypnosis was in such discredit that this book sold but a single copy. Liebault's surprising claims at first aroused considerable criticism in scientific circles, particularly from Dr. Hippolyte-Marie Bernheim, Professor of Psychiatry at Nancy.

HIPPOLYTE-MARIE BERNHEIM

Initially, Bernheim was of the opinion that Liebeault was a quack, unscientific and making false claims regarding his therapeutic successes. He resolved that it was his duty to expose Liebeault and began an investigation in order to make this exposure a thoroughly scientific one. When Liebeault cured a case of sciatica which Bernheim had treated in vain for six months, he resolved to seriously test hypnotherapy on patients.

After observing Liebeault's method and the results obtained by him on actual patients, Bernheim himself was won over to the use of hypnosis. He then began an intensive investigation over a period of years into the psychological dynamics and clinical applications of hypnosis. It was Bernheim who first recognized the great significance of the verbal suggestion employed by Liebeault. Because of his critical scientific approach, his extensive clinical studies contributed much towards a better understanding of the dynamics and mechanisms involved in hypnotic suggestion. It was he, also, who first actually demonstrated that this phenomenon of suggestion he had originally described was the real underlying factor in hypnosis; further that hypnosis was due exclusively to psychological rather than physical causes, thus disproving the original conclusions of Mesmer, Braid, Charcot and others. He established hypno-

tism as undoubtedly the most important form of psycho-
therapy of that day when he published his significant work,
Suggestive Therapeutics, in 1886. (H. Bernheim, *Suggestive
Therapeutics,* New York, Putnam. English Translation.)

CHARCOT

In 1878, J. M. Charcot began to investigate hypnosis. Charcot was already famous and highly respected for his outstanding contributions in neurology and the diseases of the
spinal cord. He studied primarily severe cases of hysteria
which had been hospitalized at the Salpetriere.

His clinical results with these cases were considered
phenomenal, and highly impressed his colleagues and students. Since he discovered that hysterical symptoms could
be either removed or created by hypnosis, he came to the
conclusion that hypnosis must be etiologically related to
hysteria and that only patients suffering from hysteria could
be hypnotized. This contention of Charcot's was later thoroughly disproved by Bernheim. Charcot was not easily convinced, and for a number of years a bitter controversy
raged between Charcot's Paris group and the Nancy school
headed by Bernheim. It appears also that Charcot did not
realize that the hypnotic influence was exercised by means
of suggestion; rather he believed that physical phenomena
were involved. For instance, on one occasion, Charcot presented a man whom he believed was quite deaf, in the
hypnotic state. He then announced that a magnet would
produce a certain effect. Bernheim then demonstrated that
the effect was due purely to the suggestion and not magnetic force; that the subject could hear perfectly well and
that a wooden imitation "magnet" produced the same remarkable effect. All past attempts to understand hypnosis
in terms of physical forces (i.e., Mesmer) or neurophysio-

logical processes (Elliotson, Charcot, Braid) had failed. The results of these investigations (Bernheim, Janet) tended more firmly to establish the significance of functional psychological factors and their role in emotional disorders, giving the organicists their first major setback.

JANET

Pierre Janet was one of the first to attempt to explain the phenomenon of hypnosis itself. He believed that the hypnotic state resulted from a progressive dissociation which occurred during hypnotic induction. He stated the view that when the conscious mind was suppressed and inhibited, the subconscious came more and more to expression; and that during deep hypnosis the subconscious finally took over completely. He felt that hypnotic phenomena and dissociation as well as certain pathological functional states (neurosis, hysteria, psychosis) were due primarily to the progressive dissipation and exhausting of psychic energy.

Janet's penetrating mind recognized certain parallels between the conscious dissociation which occurred in neurotic—and even more markedly—in psychotic states. Just as the unconscious of the psychotic becomes conscious, so the patient's subconscious, as Janet termed it, could become conscious during hypnosis.

BREUER

Through remarkable coincidence, Pierre Janet and Joseph Breuer simultaneously recognized the significance of liberating "strangulated affect" associated with traumatic experiences by means of hypnosis. This discovery of Janet and Breuer eventually proved to be of great significance in the treatment of traumatic neurosis. Later, more effective techniques for regressing patients under hypnosis and narcohypnosis were developed in order to facilitate the recall and reliving of traumatic experiences. These methods were employed effectively on a mass scale during World War II. Of interest in this regard was the excellent work of Erickson and Kubie, who applied the technique of hypnotic regression in the treatment of depression. Lindner, Grinker, Wolberg and others have made significant contributions in this area as well.

FREUD

Sigmund Freud, even as a medical student, became interested in hypnotism after witnessing the cure of a case of hysteria by his friend, Dr. Joseph Breuer. Not long afterwards, Freud decided to go to France to study hypnosis under Charcot, Berhneim and Liebeault. At first he was quite enthusiastic about what he saw. Freud, both by inclination and training, was a highly analytical and critical scientist. Although very much impressed with certain of the therapeutic accomplishments of hypnosis, he was markedly disturbed by the fact that it was not possible for him to hypnotize all of his patients. He attempts to sum up his reasons for deciding to give up the use of hypnosis in his work, *The Origin and Development of Psychoanalysis,* 1937 (L. and V. Woolf), by stating:

"When I discovered that in spite of all my efforts, I could not hypnotize by any means all of my patients, I resolved to give up hypnotism."

That he chose to discuss this matter in the above work may be significant. From his studies of hypnosis, Freud had derived considerable stimulation and new insights into the dynamics of the unconscious. In the hypnotized patient, he was able to clearly observe the phenomena of repression and transference. He was able to see how repressed memories and experiences could be recaptured by means of association while a patient was in a hypermnestic state. He was able to observe directly the intense affective reactions of the unconscious in the phenomena of abreaction and catharsis. Bernheim's experiments in which he was able to resolve what appeared to be complete posthypnotic amnesia by means of persistent questioning even in the wakeful state, impressed Freud deeply. It was after this that he speculated about the possibility of recapturing repressed memories by utilizing free association and dream analysis in the conscious state. These conclusions of Freud were of the utmost significance in the development of psychoanalysis.

In a work published in 1895, "Studien uber Hysterie," Freud and Breuer conclude, "We found at first to our greatest surprise, that the individual hysterical symptoms immediately disappeared without returning if we succeeded in thoroughly awakening the memories of the causal process with its accompanying affect, and if the patient circumstantially discussed the process in the most detailed manner and gave verbal expression to the affect." Breuer and Freud then concluded that hysterical symptoms developed as the result of the repression of painful and traumatic experiences. It seems highly probable that had not young Sigmund Freud first witnessed the treatment of that case of hysteria by Breuer and, as a result, gone to France to study hypnosis—psychoanalysis may never have been born. Furthermore, can it be that Sigmund Freud, an organically trained physician, as a result first recognized the significance of functional psychodynamics? There is no doubt that he was originally influenced by the work of Janet and Bernheim.

It is understandable that Freud because of his own personality and training, which was primarily in organic medicine, found it very difficult to accept any methods that could not be clearly and logically interpreted. He appeared to frown on active methods. Freud rejected religion for very much the same reasons. He could not tolerate anything that smacked of mysticism and metaphysics, and could not accept anything on faith. Hence he was unable to accept phenomena based on suggestion. Certainly, at the time Freud failed to realize fully the therapeutic possibilities of hypnotherapy; but that he maintained an interest for many years in hypnosis is attested to by the fact that the personal library which he left behind contained most of the significant books on the subject published during that period. In his later years, Freud admitted that if psychotherapy was ever to become widely available to the public, a return to hypnotism as a short-cut procedure would be necessary (*Collected Papers of Sigmund Freud,* Vol. 2, 1924–1925, London: Hogarth Press).

One wonders why in view of Freud's concern over the impracticability of treating large numbers of patients by psychoanalysis, that he should not have initiated and supported the study of more practical and effective methods of dealing with such needs. Was he like Adler concerned with psychotherapy for the many as well as for the few? It was already evident that an average orthodox psychoanalysis might require from three to five years, or longer. Certainly the clinical experiences of World War I and its aftermath could not have failed to impress him deeply in this respect.

Did it occur to Freud that certain of his principal objections could have been resolved by the combined use of hypnosis and psychoanalysis in the form of hypnoanalysis? Could it be that he was not fully aware of the therapeutic advantages to be gained by combining these techniques, i.e., in the facilitation and speeding up of the establishment of rapport and transference, hypermnesia and the consequent better recall, and the furthering of communication of repressed memories and fantasies, the markedly increased affective tone and prompt abreaction of patients, etc., and in the rapid uncovering of resistances and defense. Furthermore, Freud failed to exploit the great therapeutic value of consciously ventilating repressed emotional traumas after the patient emerges from the trance. (I have found, as have others, that this procedure can considerably shorten psychoanlytic therapy.)

Freud's criticism of hypnotherapy appeared to be based primarily on failures to achieve lasting cures in hysterical patients by hypnotic suggestion. He came to the conclusion that the basic cause of the patient's pathology had to be analyzed and uncovered before a permanent cure could be obtained. Certainly this makes sense; however, could not have hypnoanalysis been used more effectively toward these ends, since, as aforementioned, it so greatly facilitated the communicability and recollection of patients such that the basic causes of their illness could be more rapidly revealed. Freud later attached less significance to the conclusions of Janet and Breuer concerning the role of "strangulated affect" of early traumatic experience as the principal cause of neurosis. He became more and more impressed with the purposeful nature of symptoms, and in 1926 altered his concept of neurosis radically, expressing the view that symptoms not only represented manifestations of repressed instinctual strivings but that they also represented reaction formations and defenses against these strivings. These were therefore mechanisms to reduce or eliminate anxiety. In pointing out that symptoms often serve a purposeful and useful function in the psychic life of the patient, Freud cast considerable doubt on the value of hypnosis for the removal of symptoms. Yet somehow Freud failed to recognize the secondary as well as the immediate therapeutic benefit derived by the patient in the rapid resolution of such destructive symptoms as impotence, frigidity, etc.

Certainly Freud's contention that every patient cannot be successfully hypnotized is true. Yet, by proper application of technique some medical hypnotists achieve up to 95 per cent success, even in initial inductions. It is, however, as we all know, further clear that not every patient can be successfully analyzed. Every psychotherapeutic method presents certain advantages and disadvantages which have to be weighed, and often there are specific indications justifying the preference of one method over another. Freud referred to the strong influence of hypnotic suggestion and the power that was thereby placed in the hands of the hypnotist. He warned that one might do harm with such a powerful influence if it were not properly utilized. This is true beyond question. It is of interest that Freud, himself, had a very authoritarian approach to psychotherapy. To what extent his observations of hypnotic transference and the effect of the ominpotent authority of the hypnotist he observed, as demonstrated by Charcot on the hypnotized patient, was responsible for this attitude, is not entirely clear. Freud and his disciples centered their attack mainly on what they felt was the dependency relationship created between the hypnotist and the patient, comparing this to the role of the father to the child. This is well founded. However, have not psychoanalysts including Freud himself, repeatedly pointed to the extent of dependency and father-son transference occurring between the therapist and patient during psychoanalysis? Certainly, this may be therapeutically beneficial in many instances. Dependency feelings occur with every psychotherapeutic procedure. However, the degree of dependency fostered in a patient depends not only upon the techniques employed or the skill of the therapist and the kind of transference he creates, but upon the patient's as well as the therapist's own desires for a dependency relationship. Freud was of the opinion that patients remained improved under hypnotherapy only as long as they remained on good terms with the doctor. Thus, they felt obliged to become dependent since their dependency was the condition for their improvement. He further pointed out that the transference between the patient and the doctor had not been analyzed. Let us concede that these are true—but are these not the requirements necessary for successful psychotherapy generally; that a positive rapport and transference prevail between the patient and the doctor? In a properly conducted hypnoanalysis every effort is made to analyze the transference relationship and dependency feelings existing between the patient and therapist, and to modify these in the best interests of the therapy. Hypnoanalysis attempts to interpret the meaning of symptoms and behavior in terms of defenses and reaction formations.

For the most part, there were, of course, other reasons why hypnosis fell into clinical disrepute. The empirical rather than scientific approach by Mesmer resulted in much scepticism and disapproval among scientists. Mesmer's and later even Charcot's overenthusiastic claims, faulty conclusions, and lack of comprehension of the actual intrapsychic mechanisms operating within his hypnotized patients resulted in inestimable damage to the cause of medical hypnosis. The public began to regard it with an admixture of awe, fear, curiosity, and amusement. The medical profession at large shunned it for fear that it might discredit them.

Certainly most of the resistance to clinical hypnosis was primarily due to the sad fact that so little was known and understood about the actual nature and dynamic processes of hypnosis. It was clinical research with hypnosis that first provided clues regarding the tremendous influence of psyche over soma, and how affective disturbances could result in a physical symptom while the patient was in the hypnotic trance; i.e., Forel's induction of burn blisters and the removal of warts by Block, Swich and McDowell through hypnotic suggestion. Less dramatic but of medical interest is the fact that the author has succeeded in reducing and even eliminating inflammatory reactions such as encountered in thrombophlebitis, herpes zoster neuritis and urticaria by means of hypnotic suggestion.

In spite of all the prevailing bias, important research in hypnosis continued. Time and space do not permit the mention of all those medical scientists who bravely and determinedly conducted clinical research in hypnosis, often in the face of marked resistance and adverse criticism. Courageous investigators such as Elliotson, Braid, Liebeault, Esdaille, Bernheim, Janet, Prince, Sidis, Forel, Moll, Bianchi, Bechterev, Bramwell, Brooks, Baudouin, Yellowlees, DuBois, and many others carried the torch in spite of critical lay and professional prejudice.

Hypnosis was not only responsible in some measure for the birth of Freudian psychoanalysis, but provided direct support and impetus for our modern conception of psychosomatic medicine. By means of hypnosis, definite evidence was revealed demonstrating how psychic influences could both produce and alleviate such symptoms as headache, nausea, vomiting, asthma, gastric pain, hyperacidity, various skin disorders including urticaria, herpes, lichen ruberplanus, certain eczemas, pruritis and many other conditions.

In spite of voluminous and often brilliant research confirming the value of medical hypnosis, the rejection of its practice by the medical profession at large continued during the first half of this century and seriously hampered further research efforts and its application as an established clinical discipline. Without a doubt the insights Freud gained through hypnosis first led to the development of basic psychoanalytic theory. The advent of psychoanalysis pushed hypnosis into the background. Psychoanalysis was first promoted at the expense of excessive and discrediting attacks on hypnosis and the hypnotherapists. It was not until such recent farsighted, imaginative investigators as Erickson, Van Pelt, Wolberg, Meares, Kline, Kroger and others, conducted innumerable successful clinical investigations, that the great value of hypnosis in modern medicine was definitely established. These men must be regarded among the vanguard along with the earlier investigators, who struggled to revive and develop further one of the oldest and most effective of the healing arts into a scientific discipline and into an important clinical research technique. In addition to its use in psychotherapy, today clinical hypnosis is also being successfully applied in the fields of obstetrics, gynecology, anaesthesia, dentistry, dermatology, internal medicine and other areas. Who could have foreseen that the same British Medical Association which had discredited and rejected the work of men like the distinguished physician, Elliotson, would finally be the first to officially accept and endorse the use of hypnotic technique in medicine. Mesmer and Bernheim represent two remarkable contrasts, the former highly imaginative, bold, persuasive, creative, spectacular, brilliant and somewhat impulsive, the latter reserved, analytical, logical, cautious, patient, objective and scientifically dedicated. In their own way both these men with their particular gifts were historically indispensable and monumental figures in furthering the advance of therapeutic hypnosis. The brilliant imaginative genius of Mesmer complemented the calm objective scientific evaluation and investigation of Bernheim. It was through the latter that hypnosis first gained acceptance in medical and scientific circles as a healing art.

Chapter 2

CHARACTERISTICS OF THE HYPNOTIC STATE

THE NATURE OF HYPNOSIS

Innumerable investigations have been made in efforts to explain hypnosis on both a clinical and theoretical basis. Although some investigators like Janet, Bernheim, Pavlov and others have advanced hypothetical theories, reflecting some points of accord, on the whole there has been considerable disagreement regarding the true nature of hypnosis. Charcot and his co-workers believed that hypnotic susceptibility was a condition principally found in patients suffering from hysteria and as such could be regarded as a manifestation of the hysteric state. One of Charcot's main arguments to support this view was that hysterical patients were peculiarly susceptible to hypnosis and could be effectively treated by means of hypnotherapy, often with spectacular therapeutic results. No doubt Charcot's conclusions stemmed largely from the fact that his observations were apparently made almost exclusively on hysterical patients.

As a result of his own scepticism and interest in Liebeault's work, Bernheim undertook an intensive study of hypnotic phenomena and was able to demonstrate errors in Charcot's conclusions. For example, Bernheim discovered that hypnotic susceptibility does not necessarily require a pathological state such as hysteria, since a high percentage of normal people can be hypnotized. He found it true, however, that hysterical patients were particularly susceptible to hypnosis.

Five general concepts were advanced by investigators in attempts to account for the phenomenon of hypnosis: (1) the psychopathological concept of Charcot; (2) physiological theories offered by Heidenhain, Bennett, Vincent, Sidis, Eysenck, Hart, and others; (3) the psychophysiological theory of Pavlov; (4) the psychological suggestion concept of Bernheim, Janet, Prince, and others; (5) the atavistic regression theory of Meares.

Heidenhain thought that hypnosis resulted from inhibition of the ganglion cells of the brain. Bennett and Vincent suggested that the phenomenon was due primarily to neurophysiological alterations in the brain, such as selective inhibition of parts of the brain with overactivity of other areas. There exists clinical support for this view. Sidis speculated on a functional dissociation between the nerve cells. The primary cause of hypnosis was attributed to cerebral anemia by Hart. Eysenck believed that hypnosis was the result of selective changes at the neural junction. All of these theories, however, were largely speculative and without adequate scientific foundation.

The psychophysiological explanation of hypnosis offered by Pavlov was primarily a functional one and did not adequately stress the significance of suggestion and psychological factors.

Bennett's and Vincent's conceptions of selective cortical inhibition occurring in the hypnotic state are in substantial agreement with Pavlov. Schilder was similarly of the opinion that this selective inhibition of certain brain areas explained the "partial sleep" or "sleep vigil" in the hypnotic state. It is apparent that in hypnosis certain areas of the brain are asleep while others are in the waking state. These investigators generally leaned toward the Meares concept that hypnosis represented a form of primitive sleep and atavistic regression.

Hypnosis certainly appears to follow the sleep pattern of the higher vertebrates and primitive man. Soldiers exposed to continuous danger may develop a capacity to control their sleep depth unconsciously. For example, a Marine officer whom I hypnotized had spent three years in the South Pacific engaged in jungle warfare. Initially he was able to enter into only a light hypnotic trance. Obviously he had been conditioned to sleep lightly and to awaken easily. If Pavlov's concept of the defensive nature of hypnoidal sleep is correct, then is seems reasonable to assume that muscle reflex function remains unimpaired so the animal can act defensively when an emergency arises. Primitive man was almost constantly threatened as animals are, and had to develop these psychophysiological reactions in order to survive. That this phenomenon is not uncommon is apparent as, for example, a patient who would awaken at almost the precise moment so that she could make an early train.

In the hypnotic trance we see evidence of marked intellectual inhibitions and some dissociation as well as motoric inhibition. On the other hand, there is reduction in emotional control and inhibition with a corresponding heightened degree of affectivity and abreaction. This suggests that in the hypnotic state the individual is relieved to a considerable degree of the cultural, moral, and ethical restraints and taboos which he has acquired in the process of becoming civilized. His repressive mechanisms are largely lifted, and he is able to pour out more primitive, intense, and at times even savage and barbaric feelings.

Bernheim, Janet, Prince and others believed that the hypnotic state was primarily a psychological phenomenon because of the importance of rapport and suggestibility in hypnotic induction. Janet favored the theory of dissociation to explain hypnosis and believed that a memory or group of memories could be split off from the main stream of consciousness and give rise to a sort of second personality so that when the conscious mind was suppressed, the subconscious came more and more to the fore, and that during deep hypnosis the subconscious finally takes over completely. Van Pelt expresses the opinion that amnesia would have to be an essential factor if Janet's explanation of the trance is to be accepted. However, he points out that although amnesia frequently follows a deep trance, it is by no means constant and even when present can easily be removed by suggestion. Further, he adds that experience shows that consciousness is retained in the hypnotic state and complete control is not relinquished to the subconscious. Pavlov's concept that a cortical state of inhibition is found in hypnosis is demonstrated by experimental evidence that marked signs of both motor and psychic inhibition prevail, such as loss of spontaneous and volitional reaction, immobility, catalepsy, hypotonia, and reduced reasoning and critical, as well as discriminatory functions. Certain manifestations of subcortical, midbrain activity (phylogenetically older areas of the brain) become manifest, in particular hyperaffectivity, as well as the aforementioned.

Certain aspects of Janet's disassociation theory, Pavlov's psychophysiological theory and Meares' atavastic regression concept come closest to my own conclusions. Certainly disassociation and regression occur in the hypnotic state. Janet and Meares at least have presented a functional dynamic hypothesis of the nature of hypnosis.

My own hypothesis is based on both psychological and electrophysiological evidence that the "stream of consciousness" appears to be maintained by three primary factors—(1) the continuous stream of sensory impulses to the sensory cortex coming through our organs of perception and (2) the vast network of associative functions continuously interreacting in the human cortex and producing the phenomenon of wakeful consciousness and awareness of the external world. (3) The varying stimuli, i.e., alterations in light, color, sound, form, smell, touch, etc., produce reactions, thus contributing to consciousness and awareness.

At this point I would like to advance the thesis that when a strong, focal nonvarying stimulus is used, as for example, hypnotic fixation on a particular object, it tends to reduce and inhibit the associative processes in the sensory cortex, promoting dissociation and diminishing motor tonus and activity through an inhibitory effect on the cortex. I attribute this phenomenon to my theory of perceptual and affective priority and dominance that prevails in cortical function. Certain perceptual stimuli inhibit other awareness processes as a specific affect, i.e., rage can inhibit fear or guilt awareness. The suppressive, repressive and censoring cortical functions are reduced, furthering the release and catharsis of pent up conflict and emotion. Further, that intense concentrated fixation of a single sensory organ upon a nonvarying stimulus, tends to reduce and inhibit the perception of stimuli through other sensory organs, thereby rapidly diminishing and narrowing the field of awareness. Our sensory and psychic functions are basically comparative in organization. Neurologically, man is so functionally organized that his consciousness and critical-analytical faculties are maintained only by the continuous bombarding of the cortex with varying and therefore comparable sensory impulses, values and ideas. One can well equate change with life, nonchange with death and nothingness. I have found, experimentally, that monotonous, nonvarying stiumli facilitate corticopsychic dissociation, inhibition, regress and suggestibility. In addition to concentration on a persistent nonvarying stimulus, the major factor in hypnotic induction is that of suggestion. Thus it appears that specific repetitive types of focal stimulation result in varying degrees of intellectual and motor cortical inhibition, facilitating a marked reduction in the stream of consciousness increasing suggestibility and intensifying the trance-like state of hypnosis. *The degree of suggestibility is to a large extent dependent on the extent to which intellectual, discriminatory functions are reduced.*

A fourth factor of significance in induction of the hypnotic trance is that of verbal suggestion in the suggestive associative power of the word. Braid had originally demonstrated that a trance could be induced by, for example, optic fixation, that is, the concentration of a sensory organ on a fixed, persistent stimulus, and it was Liebault who first demonstrated that the hypnotic induction could be facilitated by means of verbal suggestion together with the Braid procedure. It is obvious that a favorable relationship between the hypnotist and his patient renders the latter more susceptible to verbal suggestion. Furthermore, the authority which the hypnotist commands in the eyes of his subject is also of considerable importance.

Andrew Salter believes that Pavlov and Beckterew were correct in regarding hypnosis as a type of conditioned response in which the suggestive associative power of the word can evoke psychophysical changes which they regard as involves conditioned reflex mechanisms. Salter points out that each time the patient is inducted into hypnosis, he becomes more susceptible as a result of the deepening of the conditioned response (akin to phenomena of dressage). Salter further points out how hypnotic suggestion heightens associative responses.

There is no doubt that the conditioned response mechanism can play an important part in hypnosis and hypnotherapy. There is no doubt that much of human behavior is of a habitually patterned sometimes rather complex pattern of response. Behavior as Salter correctly believes, is learned and once it is learned it becomes relegated to a subcortical automated type of response, i.e., we learn to drive a car consciously with effort. Later, we can talk to a friend while driving effortlessly through heavy traffic.

It is my belief that hypnotic induction is initiated by a mental or physical change which when called to the subject's attention sets off a progressive chain reaction in which the subject becomes increasingly more suggestible as suggestions are continued and changes are observed. For example, a young man suffering from a stubborn nonresponsive reaction to psychotherapy in the case of impotence was given niacin (500 mgs) with the suggestion that this would cause a wave of warmth throughout his body indicative of a sexual hormonal surge which would engorge his penis and lead to a powerful and sustained erection, whereupon he would enjoy delightful sexual fulfillment with his girlfriend. The therapeutic result was excellent. He noted that the wave of warmth he experienced convinced him that what had been suggested would occur. He felt steps of the suggested effects occurring in sequence.

Psychic Manifestations of the Hypnotic State

The hypnotic state must be regarded as a partial sleep, as a limited and altered form of consciousness, and is characterized principally by less volition and spontaneity and increased immobility. Feelings of drowsiness are also characteristic of this state. Drowsiness increases as the trance deepens. Subjective giddiness is often noted in patients when they are awakening from the trance.

Hypnotic regression to more infantile levels of reaction is partly due to reduction in time orientation sense, and is accompanied by a lessening of conscious psychic functions indicative of selective cortical inhibition. On the other hand, in the hypnotic trance, certain focal areas can react with even greater intensity when specifically stimulated, resulting in markedly increased capacity for recollection (hypermnesia). Affective reactions are likewise intensified, characteristic of earlier infantile levels of response when repressive and associative functions were not yet adequately developed. I believe that the amnestic difficulties encountered following the hypnotic trance are based on two factors primarily—the inhibition or cortical associative activity and repression of disturbing or painful material as occurs in the forgetting of dreams often soon after awakening.

As indicated, age and time regression may readily occur in the hypnotic trance upon repeated suggestion. In this regressed state the patient may actually relive his past experiences, often with considerable emotional intensity. He can be regressed back to particular periods and episodes of them as though he were a child at the respective age level at which the trauma occurred (revivification). He reacts with the emotions of a child. He may under suggestion regress to childlike handwriting and speech corresponding to the age level the subject is regressed to. This reliving of traumatic episodes may greatly facilitate recall and recollection and be of great therapeutic benefit. In the hypnotic state time distortion is a common phenomenon. Like the person experiencing a dream, the individual has little capacity to evaluate the span of time which has elapsed.

Dissociation is generally associated with regression. The hypnotized individual has not only regressed to a more primitive form of animal sleep but reacts affectively more like primitive archaic man, impulsive-compulsively and obsessively, without much exercise of foresight, critical reason, logic, or appraisal of reality. The atavistic regression theory of Meares is here worthy of consideration. He presents clinical evidence to support his view and feels that greater clinical insight into the dynamics and application of hypnosis can be attained through this hypothesis.

Since the intellectual, critical and reasoning and repressive functions are reduced and affectivity increased in the hypnotic state (hyperaffectivity), it appears logical that patients would not be able to as effectively offer resistance to analysis and would thus be better able to release repressed affect-laden conflicts. The increased degree of hypnotic transference which usually occurs, in my opinion, can be effectively employed to facilitate identification and the incorporation of feelings, thoughts, values and traits, i.e., the therapist, who in the transference may fulfill a surrogate parental role.

Freud believed that the peculiar susceptibility of the subject to give up control over his volition and action to the hypnotist was due to an unconscious desire on his part for libidinal gratification. Freud's co-worker, Ferenczi, added that hypnosis was a reactivation of the patient's infantile attitude of blind faith and implicit obedience based on both the love and fear of the parents. He further believed that the success of the hypnotist was dependent not only on the extent of transference but also upon his prestige as an all-powerful father or authority in the eyes of the patient. It is interesting that, although Freud and many of his followers were critical of the strong authoritative approach to the patient they nevertheless incorporated the "prestige" approach in their psychoanalytical rituals. According to Freud, the analyst had to be strong and secure and inspire respect for his position. In fact, the analyst must be so strong, pure, and incorruptible as not to be susceptible to most of the moral weaknesses of men, a kind of therapeutic priesthood. He should attain the acme of objectivity.

Of particular interest, are certain alterations in the psychic functions occurring in the hypnotic state. For instance, there is a marked ability to fantasize and hallucinate. As Schilder pointed out, the hypnotized subject's perceptual world is altered. He sees things others do not, and he does not see things others do. The mere command of the hypnotist can arouse new and vividly colorful images before him. This particular enhanced ability to project artistic images is beautifully exploited in the hypnography technique employed by Meares. By means of suggestion, objects can be distorted in size and form or color (perceptual illusion).

This interesting phenomenon of the hypnotic state is that of being able to induce sensory perceptual alterations, as for example with regard to time, gustatory, olfactory, and body image distortions. These perceptual alterations can occur in hypnotic suggestion as well as in posthypnotic suggestion.

In the past, I have noted that several of my patients who had to undergo open heart surgery were quite fearful of the so-called "cooling the body" down procedure. Concerned about this I considered the possibility of creating a "thermal illusion effect." One beautiful day at our ocean beach, I found the opportunity. It was a bright sunny day. The skies were blue and all was perfect except that the water temperature was 57° Fahrenheit and not a single person was in the water. I got together 15 young adult volunteers and hypnotized them as a group. I then gave them posthypnotic suggestions that they would upon awakening from the trance, go into the water and find the temperature delightful. They would first feel some tingling and a slight burning of the skin but this would be due to the initial contact with the water: that this effect would be due to the warmth of the water. Soon after the initial sensation they would feel like they were in tropical water in Florida. They would feel delightfully comfortable and would play and frolic and even splash each other as though they were kids again in a warm bathtub.

The induction was completely successful, and upon awakening from the trance, the group immediately went into the water in line, duck fashion. The group was enjoying themselves thoroughly and had been in the water about 15 minutes when the captain of the beach patrol rushed up with a jeep, alarmed, believing that the subjects were in the water in a hypnotized state. Further, he was angry because the group had gone in between the life guard stations. He ordered the guards to bring the people out because they didn't want to come out voluntarily. They were enjoying themselves too much. A large crowd gathered and looked on with amusement and amazement. The *Atlantic City Press* carried a headline, "Washington Psychiatrist Turns North Atlantic into Caribbean."

As aforementioned, the general background in terms of education, intelligence, culture, religion, family and life experience, is a contributing factor determining the degree of suggestibility. Some individuals manifest a high degree of suggestibility (hypersuggestibility) prior to hypnotic induction. Such individuals are obviously easily hypnotized. As a result of repeated hypnotic induction, it is possible to make individuals increasingly suggestible—the phenomenon of dressage. This high degree of suggestibility may not only be manifest during the hypnotic trance, but also in the posthypnotic state, and is often of value in hypnotherapy. Increased suggestibility may be selective in terms of autosuggestibility, as distinguished from a high degree of suggestibility to external suggestion. In most instances the highly suggestible patient is readily influenced by both auto and external suggestion.

At this point a word of caution is appropriate. It is generally not advisable in certain instances to foster a too marked degree of suggestibility, since this may result in some instances in undersirable complications such as the spontaneous trance. This is particularly so with patients who tend to be withdrawn, introverted, autistic, with tendencies toward fantasies and escapism.

Hypnotic suggestion can markedly heighten the anticipatory state of the patient. A patient who anticipates a certain influence or effect upon himself is more likely to manifest increased suggestibility. Furthermore, each suggestive influence which the patient experiences in himself intensifies and augments further response to suggestion (chain response). Posthypnotic suggestion may greatly enhance anticipatory feelings. The great importance of certain symbolic gestures in enhancing the suggestibility of the patient is well expressed by Meares in his discussion of the atavistic regressive character of induction of the hypnotic state. Meares, for example, stresses that a simple suggestion is more likely to be accepted by the patient and that as this is accepted, the patient will respond progressively to more complex suggestions. This is also indicative of the chain reaction pattern of suggestibility.

Suggestibility can be enhanced by sedative, anaesthetics and alcohol, drugs which sedate the ego and the reality-testing capacities (narcohypnosis). Furthermore, suggestibility can be increased by rhythmic movements, by repetitive sounds, by fatigue, and other factors. We must recognize that hypnotic suggestion is more perceptive than intellectual, and is emotionally charged, and therefore tremendously influenced by the affective relationship between the patient and the therapist. It is for this reason that appeals to logic, to reason, to step-by-step analysis and evaluation do not increase suggestibility, but generally lessen it, because they tend to awaken the critical faculties of the mind and to activate the reality-testing capacities.

Suggestibility is enhanced when there is emotional security and absence of threat. A close relationship between the patient and therapist makes sharing of feelings and beliefs easier. Also suggestibility is increased when the therapist speaks with authority and utters monotonous, repetitive words. I have also found experimentally that suggestibility can be greatly enhanced by exposing the patient to authoritative confirmation of the therapist's observations by others. I term this "auxiliary suggestion."

Somnambulism or "waking hypnosis" is characterized by the absence of sleep manifestations such as drowsiness and immobility. The individual is wide awake. He is consciously aware of what is transpiring around him. He is, however, in a highly suggestible state and may manifest hypnotic phenomena such as catalepsy, hyperreflexia, varying degrees of anaesthesia, functional paralysis and, on suggestion, catatonic type bodily rigidity may often be induced. This state bears a resemblance to what is commonly referred to as "sleep walking." Although the patient is wide awake his reasoning and logical faculties are reduced. It has been demonstrated experimentally by Erikson and others that, in this state, subjects, when put under marked pressure, will generally act to preserve their security and to protect themselves, as, for example, if a somnambulist receives a suggestion that he will commit a homicidal act or commit a robbery. If the command is in marked conflict with his moral ethics, the individual will resist or may even awaken from the somnambulistic trance. Because of the character of the somnambulistic state, it is entirely possible, even for an expert hypnotist to sometimes overlook the fact that the patient is in a trance. Since somnambulistic states may occur spontaneously in patients who have been repeatedly hypnotized, it is wise to guard against this eventuality and to from time to time test the state of the patient.

Of great importance in hypnotherapy is the phenomena of posthypnotic suggestion. If the individual is given a specific command that he will carry out a particular act at a given time in the future, he may execute this command in a manner that appears to be an automatic compliance, unaware, he is carrying out a command which has been planted in his subconscious mind. The extent to which he will comply depends on the degree of resistance he feels toward the particular command, or the hypnotist giving him the command. Compliance depends also on whether he is a highly defensive, competitive or cooperative personality. Further, of importance is the authority and forcefulness employed by the suggestor. It has been demonstrated experimentally by such workers as Erikson and others, that an individual will not likely carry out an act under posthypnotic suggestion which threatens his own personal security or represents a serious legal or moral violation. Posthypnotic suggestion can, for instance, be used not only to create an artificial amnesia, but to further recall, recollection and fantasy. Posthypnotic suggestion has been employed to relieve pain and to induce sleep. I have found it to be of great value in the treatment of impotence, frigidity and other sexual problems. It is of great value in symptom removal or reduction. Its place in hypnotherapy will be discussed at length later.

PHYSICAL MANIFESTATIONS OF THE HYPNOTIC STATE

By suggestion of the hypnotist marked somatic changes can occur, particularly in those parts of the body which are innervated by the vegetative nervous system. Thus, in the trance, the hypnotist can produce bodily changes which the subject could not willfully create or alter. Since affectivity, as indicated earlier, is increased in the hypnotic trance, such somatic effects occur as a result of intensified emotional reaction, i.e., vasomotor constriction or dilation, slowing or speeding of the heart or respiration, gastrointestinal secretion and motility, disphoresis and pupillary changes, etc. Experimentally, Forel, Schultz, Heller, and Alrutz have even elicited burn blisters by means of hypnosis. I had occasion to observe that hypnotic suggestion tended to reduce the inflammatory reaction in thrombophlebitis of the lower extremities. That hypnosis can influence the menstrual cycle is well-known. I have found that hypnotic influence can create marked gastric nausea or emesis or can relieve these conditions when they exist. Hypnosis has been effectively employed by myself, i.e., in the successful treatment of a number of cases of pernicious vomiting in pregnancy.

The hypotonia of the hypnotic state is very similar to the waxy flexibility found in catatonic stupor. Bearing some similarity to this state is the cataleptic phenomena of hypnosis (catalepsy), in which the patient presents inordinate and prolonged fixed maintenance of the postures and body parts as observed in catatonic schizophrenics. One of the striking features of the hypnotic trance is the patient's state of physical immobility. This is indicative of marked inhibitory effects of the motor cortex. The cataleptic phenomena represents clear evidence of the loss of spontaneous movement. In the hypnotic trance we note further that there is an accompanying marked inhibition of the cortical motor speech center with a reduction or loss of spontaneous speech. During the trance, movement can be initiated by the hypnotist. This movement is automatic in that it is not subject to the voluntary control of the patient. The extent of the loss of voluntary motor control depends on the depth of the trance. Thus, in the hypnotic trance, prolonged automatic movement of an extremity can be achieved upon the command of the hypnotist. This phenomena, as we shall note later, can be effectively employed as a trance deepening procedure. The automatic movement can be promptly terminated by the suggestions or command of the therapist.

Of further interest is the fact that similar automation is characteristic of certain schizophrenic states, particularly in catatonics. In the hypnotic state some degree of automatic compliance and obedience is usually manifest. Schizophrenic, and in particular, catatonic patients often tend to carry out instructions of others in a blind, obedient manner often without the exercise of critical or automatic judgment. In the hypnotic trance, patients, although compliant, are capable of resisting instructions or suggestions to a limited degree, depending on the trance depth. This is particularly evident when instructions, commands or suggestions are given to the patient which, he feels, threaten or endanger his life or security.

In hypnosis, even though the muscle tone is very relaxed, we have noted that the tendon reflexes are responsive and in some instances even hyperreactive. Generally, the degree of muscle tonus varies in the hypnotic state, depending largely upon the depth of trance. This, I believe, lends support to the conclusion that in this state of hypnoidal sleep the animal or human can readily be awakened and prepared to defend himself. Further support for the hypothesis that hypnosis is a form of sleep, is the fact that patients can be readily transferred from the hypnotized state to deep sleep. Similarly, often patients who have been in autohypnosis were frequently able to pass from this state into deep sleep.

On the other hand, during the hypnotic as well as in the somnambulistic trance, it is possible to induce states of catatonic-like muscular rigidity. This latter phenomenon has often been exploited for entertainment in which a hypnotist demonstrates the unique spectacle of a person lying extended and rigid as board between two chairs. Rigidity can often become so marked that it is, for instance, impossible to bend the patient's elbow by ordinary force, and these rigid postures can be maintained for surprisingly long periods.

Of further interest is the fact that most patients have reduced pain sensation during the hypnotic trance. This analgesia-anaesthesia can be increased by means of hypnotic suggestion. It is, further, impossible to induce hyperaesthesia by means of hypnotic suggestion. The mechanism of action here appears to be either a diminished or heightened cortical awareness of pain. We shall later discuss the application of hypnosis to analgesia and anaesthesia.

During the hypnotic trance there is not only a reduction or loss of spontaneous movement and volition but also of spontaneous speech. This may vary from a partial to a complete loss of spontaneous speech. The speech generally is reduced in tone except when the patient is in an agitated state. There may be considerable hesitation in speech. Two factors are involved here, that of emotional blocking, and further, that distortion of time occurs in the hypnotic state. Of interest is the fact that intellectual processes are reduced while affectivity is enhanced. Varying degrees of amnesia can be induced depending on the trance depth. Amnesia can be produced or deepened by posthypnotic suggestion.

SLEEP AND HYPNOSIS

One of the most disputed questions is that of whether hypnosis and sleep are related mechanisms. Schilder, Pavlov and others believe hypnosis to be a form of sleep. Van Pelt believes that hypnosis and sleep are not identical. He bases his views on the following points: First, that hypnosis can be induced without any mention of sleep at all, and second, for example, he points out that a whispered suggestion which a sleeping person would ignore entirely, might be adequate to bring about a most complicated reaction if given during hypnosis. Further, he indicates that consciousness, which is entirely suspended in natural sleep, is present in the state of hypnosis, and points to the work of Bass who has demonstrated that the patellar reflex, or knee jerk, which is normally absent in sleep is present in hypnosis as in the waking state. The author has, however, found instances of patients in a medium to deep trance in whom the patellar reflex was reduced or completely absent. Van Pelt refers to the observations of Wible and Jenness who demonstrated by means of electrocardiographic and respiratory studies that the normal difference between heart and lung action in sleep and the waking state did not exist in hypnosis and that the trance state was more like normal consciousness than sleep.

Further, Loomis, Harvey and Hobart demonstrated that evoked brain potentials of subjects in a hypnotic trance were characteristic of those obtained in the waking state. In addition, Estabrooks described an experiment with the "psychogalvanic reflex" apparatus which measures skin resistance to a very small amount of electric current. This resistance changes under emotional strain and was shown to be the same in hypnosis as in the waking state unless a sleep-like condition was deliberately suggested to the subject.

According to the author's view, there is evidence that the hypnotic state, as Van Pelt points out, presents many of the characteristics of consciousness; however, there are definite manifestations which are related to sleep. Pavlov's observations concerning the cortical inhibition occurring in hypnosis cannot be underestimated. Conscious awareness in hypnosis is generally reduced, although it may be accentuated in focal cortical areas. Affective reactions in hypnosis bear a close resemblance to the affective experiences in the dream state in which there is a partial suspension of consciousness. Likewise, time distortion and age regression occur as in the dream state. Schilder points out that the behavior of a person in deep hypnosis corresponds in every detail to that of the sleeper. He quivers as he goes to sleep, he rubs his eyes as he awakens; reflex responses upon emerging from a hypnotic trance, are similar to those of a person awakening from sleep. In addition, patients often describe feelings of drowsiness, giddiness, mental cloudiness and mild confusion which take some time to dissipate, as are likewise encountered in persons awakening from sleep. He goes on to point out that more or less all shades of transition between dreaming and waking consciousness are encountered. He points out that the state of consciousness of the hypnotized subject differs from that of the sleeper in that the former maintains his contact and rapport with the hypnotist, while the sleeper does not. In final analysis, he concludes, it is merely a particular form of sleep vigil. He states that one part of the personality sleeps, or rather dreams; another is turned toward the hypnotist in the fashion of sleep vigil; still another watches lest the person undertake something, for the sake of the hypnotist, which is against his own interest.

As Schilder also points out, hypnosis is a form of "sleep vigil" in which the sleeper maintains contact and rapport with the hypnotist. It further appears, that the hypnotic trance represents a state in which elements of sleep and consciousness are present; that is, a transitional state which resembles the hypnoidal sleep of animals in which contact is not completely lost with the external world, representing a type of protective awareness and lighter sleep that exists as a defense against external dangers. This form of sleep vigil was very common among front line troops who were exposed to constant danger. When there is a constant threat, the individual generally goes through a readjustment of his sleep function, demonstrating a progressive pattern of increasingly lighter sleep and easier awakening, often awakened by merely the cracking of a twig. In these instances the brain is not totally asleep, but selectively aware, and generally hypnosis can be regarded as a form of partial primitive sleep, in which the capacity to ward off external danger is not completely lost.

Pavlov also pointed to the similarity of the hypnotic state to the hypnoidal sleep of animals in which contact is not completely lost with the external world and represents a form of sleep vigil and awareness that exists as a defense against external dangers. In my opinion, the differing views concerning whether hypnosis is a form of sleep or not are largely derived from the fact that in hypnosis certain areas of the brain are selectively inhibited and sleep while others are conscious or even hyperreactive. Thus hypnosis is somewhat similar to the dream state in which part of the brain is asleep while other areas diurnally inactive, submerged from consciouness and repressed by the waking ego, continue activity. It is interesting that individuals show considerable variability in depth of sleep and that this can often be correlated closely not only with general fatigue but with the degree of freedom from anxiety and emotional security of the particular individual.

I have noted in observing a large series of cases that insomniacs who have repeated difficulty in falling asleep, often had greater difficulty in entering a hypnotic trance. Further, a higher percentage of these subjects were refractory to hypnotic induction. This, of course, suggests that there are certain parallel conditions necessary for both sleep and hypnosis. In such cases, patients often reveal fears of loss of control, of being attacked, or of death.

The Hypnotic State

The hypnotic state is characterized by marked motoric and verbal inhibition. As the trance deepens, the individual becomes more immobile, the muscles flaccid with increasing hypotonia. The subject becomes more and more cataleptic as the trance deepens. Tendon reflexes, such as the patellar and archilles, are retained or even accentuated. As the trance progresses, there is progressively deepening drowsiness. There is marked loss of voluntary function with a disappearance of initiative and spontaneity. The subject will not usually speak but will answer if questioned. The subject beomes increasingly compliant to authority. Suggestibility is progressively heightened as the hypnotic trance deepens. Only in instances where there is still some resistance are compliance and suggestibility reduced. In such cases compliance and suggestibility may be limited. Or there may be indications of negativism; for example, when asked to raise his left hand, he raises his right hand. During the hypnotic state, the patient becomes hyperaffective, sometimes bursting out with spontaneous tears and expressions of sorrow. Although the emotional responses are heightened, the intellectual and logical reasoning processes are reduced. All conscious awareness is constricted. Concentration on the voices and instructions of the hypnotist becomes marked. There is a progressive, transitory loss of reality sense and a heightened capacity for fantasy, particularly if suggested. Therefore diurnal and noctornal dreams dealing with significant material, either in the past, the present or projected into the future, may be induced by hypnotic suggestion. Due to a progressively greater loss of time sense, regression back to earlier levels of experience is facilitated. Memory is accentuated in the hypnotic trance, no doubt in part due to lifting of repressive mechanisms as well as to be more easily able to regress back and recall earlier associations. This hypermnesia plus the enhanced capacity to regress and reexperience earlier levels contributes to enhanced phenomena for revivification—that is, intensely reliving past experiences as though they were actually occurring. It is interesting that the capacity to regress based on a loss of time sense occurs not only in the hypnotic state but in dreams.

PSYCHOSOMATIC EFFECTS

Hypnotic suggestion can produce marked physiologic changes due to its profound effect on the autonomic and vasomotor nervous system. Marked alterations in pulse rate and blood pressure can be induced. Vasomotor effects in the skin can be achieved through suggestion, i.e., reddening, urticaria and even burn blisters as was first achieved by Forel. The author induced Herpes Zoster lesions in a patient who was suffering from a localized spinal neuritis, then removed them by hypnotic suggestion in a short time and soon after reinduced them, then quickly resolved the Herpes Zoster by hypnotic suggestion for a second time. Gastrointestinal effects such as nausea, vomiting, may be readily induced by hypnotic suggestion. Hypnotic suggestion can markedly alter the pain threshold as for example, in hypnoanalgesia and hypnoanaesthesia. Muscle tone can be markedly affected and hypotonia or muscular rigidity can be induced by hypnotic suggestion. Sensory perception may be heightened or constricted. Perceptivity can be markedly increased or lessened by hypnotic suggestion.

An interesting phenomena of the hypnotic state is the heightened anticipatory state and degree of expectancy. Not only is the temporal sense reduced as in age-regression but the capacity to project into the future and visualize future achievements is often greatly enhanced. Certainly the phenomena of anticipation is present in animals who store food for the crisis of winter, etc. Likewise, primitive man could only survive by gathering food, fur, fuel, etc. Anticipatory capacities such as of the power of atomic weapons are necessary to man's survival in our current time.

Both negative and positive anticipatory reactions can be markedly intensified in the hypnotic state. This reaction can be used to therapeutic advantage as a strong, initially motivating reaction. Specifically, I used hypnosis to enhance the anticipatory reactions and foresight of offenders who had had difficulty in foreseeing the consequences of their acts. The subjects were told to fantasize a homicide under hypnosis and experience all the painful consequences. After going through such an experience, the protagonist invariably loses his desire to commit the act. No doubt, a number of potential homicides were prevented by this method.

ANTICIPATORY EFFECTS AND HYPNOSIS

It is not only what the individual anticipates and expects from others that affects him. As an individual develops, he acquires a self-image. He is either the good boy or bad, the smart one or the dumb, the hard worker or the lazy one, etc. He comes to feel that others expect a certain type of behavior from him. As cast in a play, he feels impelled to play a certain role.

Anticipatory reactions related to external events are based on earlier experience. Anticipatory reactions concerning our own future reactions often rise in our unconscious and exist there for some time before finally becoming manifest. Much of what we term "foresight" and what governs our long-range planning is certainly largely based on anticipatory functions.

Animals anticipate the winter—squirrels hoard their nuts, bees their honey, birds fly south. We have attributed many of these anticipatory reactions to instinct. If so, then instinctive reactions must be very closely related to the anticipatory function which in man we find localized in the most recently acquired part of the brain, namely, the fore-brain.

When we say "hope springs eternal in the human breast," we see how basically related human motivation is to positive anticipatory feelings which we term "hope." Most of human happiness is largely dependent on a rather regular flow of such positive anticipation in a mind that is not despairing of the future and not too morbidly preoccupied with the present.

Negative anticipation gives rise to frequently unnecessary painful anxieties, bitterness, and despondency along with phobic, hysteric and paranoid symptoms. This negative anticipation often becomes so real and disturbing to patients that they act out an imagined illness or dreaded event.

Both negative and positive anticipatory reactions can be markedly intensified in hypnosis. During the hypnotic trance, suggestion is a powerful stimulant of anticipatory reactions, feelings, and fantasies. This is, of course, due to the fact that all affective reactions are markedly increased during the hypnotic trance. Since anticipatory factors are so closely correlated to motivation, it is clear that these are often of great therapeutic significance.

There is probably no area in which anticipatory factors play as much of a role as in sexuality. A man may dread that he will not achieve or sustain an erection or that he will experience a premature ejaculation. A woman who has repeatedly failed to achieve orgasm may lose her sexual desire and come to regard the sexual act with such apprehension and despair that she is literally incapable of any normal gratifying experience. On the other hand, the man or woman who has repeatedly experienced gratification not only looks forward to the experience with anticipated pleasure but is able to relax and fully enjoy the preliminary lovemaking and foreplay. In the former instance, the individual sets up defenses against not having too painful an experience by attempting to curb sexual excitation, as for example, the woman who has been repeatedly disappointed by an impotent lover. Such a woman often does not permit herself to become very sexually excited or avoids a sexual encounter because of the apprehension of being disappointed.

For instance, I have found that the anticipatory factor is of great significance in most cases of psychic impotence or frigidity. This I have been able to confirm by administering placebos, which had been suggested to the respective patients as powerful sexual stimulants, usually while they were in a hypnotic trance. A rationale for the placebo effects was explained under hypnosis to the patient in considerable detail. In most instances, strong posthypnotic suggestion resulted not only in marked pleasurable anticipation but in virtually automatic fulfillment of the commands given resulting in adequate gratification. For instance, male patients who had been functionally partially or completely impotent were enabled to have sustained erections and gratify their partners. This initial "fait accompli" was often therapeutically decisive. Suggestibility can be strongly enhanced by giving a posthypnotic suggestion that a certain medication will produce a marked sexual reaction characterized by a wave of heat through the body and stepped up potency. The patient feeling the heat reaction induced by Niacin (500 mgs.) which I employ becomes progressively more charged in sexual desire and potency. By means of inducing the aforementioned bodily reaction which the patient experiences, a chain reaction of heightened suggestibility is established.

The results in over 90 per cent of the cases were most impressive. These patients were able to overcome their sexual impotence and frigidity and to achieve normal gratification. Once this was accomplished, patients were often able to accept themselves as sexually adequate men or women. Furthermore, they thereby gained sufficient insight to recognize their conditions as the result of emotional disturbances when they were thus convinced that their problem was functional and that they could not have been organically impaired. Once the sexual experience is genuinely gratifying, the anticipation of future similar pleasurable experiences is obvious. In fact, the positive anticipation usually continues to mount with each successful experience. A word of caution is appropriate here. Many patients will respond well to suggestion and be prepared to function well sexually but are thwarted by a rejecting, critical or unloving sex partner. When conducting hypnotherapy of sexual problems, it is highly important, when at all possible, to obtain the cooperation of sexual partners and to direct them as to their therapeutic input.

Negative anticipatory reactions may be defined as pessimism, positive anticipatory reactions as optimism. Unconscious or preconscious anticipation, it appears, is akin to a sort of intuitive reaction. In the hypnotic trance certain intuitive reactions appear to be sharpened.

I have had occasion to hypnotize numerous patients who had traveled considerable distances after receiving strong assurances that they could be helped by me. In every instance, thus far, these patients have gone into trances without any difficulty—in fact, in some instances, well nigh spontaneously. There is little likelihood of resisting what one already anticipates and desires to the extent indicated by a patient going to considerable expense and trouble to seek treatment.

Certainly a large element of suggestibility is anticipation. The anticipation of a specific effect appears to lower the hypnotic threshold. This can be readily observed on induction. The subject anticipates a similar reaction to similar stimuli. This anticipatory factor, in my opinion, plays an important role in the "conditioned response," i.e., the phenomena of dressage on hypnotic induction.

The prestige and authority of the hypnotist are greatly enhanced by positive, successful accomplishments, particularly with persons in close relationship to the patient. Furthermore, the initial anxiety of the patient is greatly relieved by the accounts given by patients already successfully treated. The confidence of the patient also frequently appears, unconsciously as well as consciously, to influence the hypnotist in such a way that he is actually more effective —persuasive, strong, and decisive.

Hypnosis provides the most effective method for studying the dynamics of anticipation. An understanding of these dynamics is of tremendous import for all successful hypnotherapy and all other forms of psychotherapy. First, we must differentiate between anticipation on the conscious level and anticipation of a subconscious (preconscious) or unconscious type. In general, anticipatory reactions relating to external events or situations are based primarily on earlier experiences. In many instances, what appears to be conscious anticipation is actually greatly influenced or motivated by unconscious anticipatory reactions. Anticipatory reactions concerning our own future responses or actions often arise in our deeper unconscious and may exist there for some time before finally becoming overtly manifest. At times they remain at a precognitive level. In the unconscious, such anticipatory reactions may often give rise to affective disturbances such as anxiety, guilt, or anger. Consciously, such emotional disturbances within the unconscious may not be manifest as a specific affective reaction, but rather as a generalized tension or irritability or in the form of physical systems. Anticipatory reactions during the hypnotic state are generally highly charged with affectivity, i.e., if an individual is in an anxious state, under hypnosis he will probably have marked dread of certain future events. Very often the unconscious ego, or superego, seeks to repress or ward off disturbing anticipatory reactions. Reaction formations are unconsciously created against the dread possibility. In addition to the signs of tension, irritability, and restlessness, psychosomatic symptoms, particularly such as sweating, rapid pulse, increased blood pressure, headache, throbbing of the temples, dizziness, and many others, may be manifest. Often behind attitudes or particular attentiveness and considerateness are concealed evidences of deeper resentment and an impulse to hurt a particular person, namely, the person who is the object of such tender consideration. It is as if the unconscious is saying, "How could I have any harmful or aggressive intent; you see how kind and considerate I am?" Most of us, at one time or another, would probably have given open expression to our resentment, in an active form, had we not thought of consequences. The anticipatory function is a very necessary social security and protective device, not only for protection against harming others, but for the protection of ourselves. In the psychoneurotic patient, there usually exists a tendency to over-exaggerate or distort both negative and positive anticipations. Destructive and negative anticipatory emotional disturbances within the individual are generally repressed to an unconscious level. By means of hypnoanalysis, it is often possible to rapidly explore these disturbed feelings. Since the individual is highly susceptible to positive suggestive influence under the hypnotic trance in each state, the anticipatory function can be highly activated. This is not only due to the increased state of affectivity but also to the heightened degree of imagination and fantasy which can be effected in the hypnotic trance.

In this connection, let us for a moment consider some of the developmental factors which influence the anticipatory process.

We see the child attempting to achieve mastery over the world around him (Mastery Instinct). He is forever testing himself. Out of this testing, he acquires an estimate of his capacities and is able gradually to determine or anticipate what he can or cannot do. If he is initially unsuccessful, he comes of course to anticipate failure. If his first attempts are successful, he looks forward with eagerness and positive anticipation to overcome the challenge. Thus, his early initial testing experiences take on added significance. Similarly, early social rejections and disappointments and hurts tend to create negative anticipatory feelings in the child. Defenses are erected against others hurting him again, and the child begins frequently to evade and avoid social contact. Such failure of acceptance and approval by others inevitably leads to feelings of inadequacy and inferiority, self-condemnation, self-rejection. This gives rise to principally two reactions within the child. Either the child develops a deep-seated feeling of defeatism (What's the use?), or despair, and a socially vicious cycle of withdrawal of interest and effort; or the child shows a completely opposite reaction and tends to exert a strong compensatory striving (I'll show them!).

It is interesting that Pavlov observed withdrawal in dogs submitted to painful or oppressive stimuli or conditions likewise. Two types of reactions—one he called inhibitory, the other excitatory—could be observed in his animals.

The "I'll show them!" child often goes to excesses to demonstrate his superiority or to convince others that he is not inferior, that he can "measure up." Measuring up is very apropos to our modern contemporary American culture. It has become a "must." Note the contempt in our society for weakness, failure, infirmity, old age, and poverty. The powerful, strong, beautiful, and rich are idealized. Most children who have built up a considerable reservoir of self-rejection and condemnation tend often to deeply resent themselves. Out of this deep inner self-resentment, the child frequently projects self-hate and externalizes this towards others in a socially hostile and destructive manner. Later an attempt shall be made to try more clearly to develop the interaction dynamics of self-hate, guilt, and hostility. Hence we can readily see that any familial, social or educational system which tends to make strong or excessive demands upon the child, to which he can hardly measure up or adhere, is a system which tends to exert a very critical or deprecatory influence and would greatly aggravate a child's feelings of inferiority, inadequacy, self-contempt, and self-hate. The greater the demands on the child, the greater are the possibilities of failure and his not measuring up. Frequently the child may resent these excessive demands and this may seriously discourage constructive motivation and initiative. In addition, excessive demands very often create unnecessary anxieties and anticipations of failure in the child. The child, unable to measure up to these excessive demands, may often feel bitterly frustrated and resentful. He may adopt the attitude in so many words of "I just can't win." Often, as a result, he develops guilt and shame feelings, for after all how often it has been pointed out to him by his teachers that other children have made the grade. How very painful this is to young Johnny! He becomes increasingly sensitive at being compared unfavorably with his peers. Although Johnny has the potentiality to measure up to the others, his self-confidence and self-esteem have been seriously affected. Such instances may be even more aggravated in cases where Johnny happens to be "a late bloomer." Certainly children greatly need motivation and drives. The reasons are manifold. Here we have not only such factors as discouragement and deprecation at home but also cultural factors such as the general background of the parents, their educational level, their ability to communicate intelligently and understandingly with their children. Of great significance too in this regard is the degree of initiative and drive which parents demonstrate, for parents are the first teachers and supply the example of the *modus operandi* for dealing with life situations. It may be too that the child has not been emotionally preconditioned to a competitive relationship with other children in a competitive society. Certainly if a child has been previously taught a cooperative attitude, then the competitive situation may present a serious conflict. As a result of Johnny's initial disturbances and failures, he all too often comes to anticipate failure. Some parents encourage strong competitiveness with children and push the child towards being a "standout," or "at the top of his class," while more accepting parents feel that a child should not be pushed but should develop naturally and be motivated by his developing interests from within and not by pressures from without.

Here we must consider whether the parent is seeking to gratify his own pride (ego) or is primarily concerned with his child's happiness.

Depth of Hypnosis

Hypnosis is a state characterized by a partial relinquishing of consciousness, with varying degrees of cortical motor and sensory inhibitions, depending upon the depth of the trance. Muscle tone can range from complete relaxation to marked rigidity and catalepsy depending upon suggestions given.

As has already been described, it resembles the light hypnoidal sleep of certain animals who have been able to survive because of their ability to awaken readily in case of danger. Similarly, the hypnotized patient is usually on guard and ready to awaken if any real threat to his security occurs. The partially conscious ego remains vigilantly on guard. In exceptional cases patients may be hypnotized into such a deep trance, usually referred to as hypnotic coma, that the defensive capacity of the ego is virtually nil. This is, however, unusual and requires strong trust and susceptibility to suggestion. Generally, there is some degree of amnesia following a deep trance. Amnesia can be deepened by posthypnotic suggestion.

The phenomena of dressage is to be noted here. Usually, the subject goes into a progressively deeper trance successively following each induction. If the subject does not go progressively deeper each time, it is generally indicative of resistance.

For practical therapeutic purposes, the deep (coma) trance is rarely necessary. Clinical studies on the therapeu-

tic value of various depths of hypnosis have been conducted by Van Pelt, Erickson, and Wolberg. The author is
generally in agreement with Van Pelt's conclusion that the
light trance is often of greater therapeutic value. Where
resistance and noncompliance are encountered, on occasion a deeper trance may be therapeutically beneficial. If
the principal aim is influencing the subject, then the light
trance would probably not be as effective. However, if the
prime purpose is psychotherapeutic and the facilitating of
understanding and meaningful communication, then the
light trance would be more advantageous. It is clear that
the greater the loss of consciousness, the greater the difficulty in recall and verbal communication. If the psyche
becomes too inhibited and clouded, there would not only
be little or no insight into the material discussed but pro-
ductivity in general would be greatly reduced. Likewise,
narcohypnosis has the disadvantage of clouding of consciousness and impairing both memory recall and intellectual associations. If the psyche is too deeply hypnotized by
drugs or by frank induction, the affective responses may be
reduced and catharsis-abreaction can be greatly lowered.

As aforementioned, I have run a number of tests in
which attempts were made to observe the reactions of subjects to several therapists with different voices. Invariably
the subject, after being introduced to a number of doctors
under hypnosis, would select the voice of a certain doctor
with whom he or she might desire to communicate. It was
further found in these tests that often such a subject would
communicate material hitherto repressed from the therapist with whom he might have been working for several
months or longer. I have found that subjects would develop
much more rapid positive transference with a therapist
whose voice they had selected as very pleasing and sympathetic. Patients under hypnosis are highly sensitive to the
attitude and feelings emanating from the therapist.

The feelings of the patient towards the therapist as

well as the general overall "affective tone" of the patient markedly affects suggestibility, hypnotic, and posthypnotic compliance.

The posthypnotic influence generally remains effective only as long as the suggestion or command remains submerged in the unconscious. The influence is generally lost when it is recalled or brought to conscious awareness. Experimentally, the author has used suggestion to help block the conscious recall of disturbing beliefs or feelings with some success. Pleasurable diversions can often be established by hypnotic suggestion.

Generally, in the hypnotic state, affectivity is greatly intensified, emotions are deeply felt, tears and joy are prompt and marked. Our affective life is inhibited, repressed, and suppressed by the conscious self operating the sensory cortex. When the conscious self is inactivated, just as in a nocturnal dream, feelings of love, passion, fear, and hate are strongly experienced.

This high degree of affectivity can be exploited therapeutically in a number of ways:

1. Marital counselling—by making possible understanding, communication, and tension release between the partners concerned.
2. Criminal investigation—in determining degree and character of emotional motivation and the state of feeling preceding the crime.
3. Catharsis and release of unbearable disturbing tensions.
4. To increase joyous and successful anticipation and thereby step up the motivation of depressed patients.
5. To increase pleasurable anticipation of orgasm in frigid and impotent patients. As pointed out, joyous anticipation is a strongly motivating force towards fulfillment.

6. Catharsis; that is, discharges of strongly repressed conflicts can be more easily effected by intensifying affective reactions. Affect is usually bound to specific conflicts when strong affective discharges occur. The related conflictual material may be likewise unburdened, somewhat in the manner of an emotional chain reaction.

Chapter 3

PREPARATION OF THE PATIENT FOR INDUCTION

Every person who seeks hypnotherapy for the first time has certain questions on his mind, i.e., "Can it hurt me? How do I know it will work? How will I know if I am hypnotized? Will I awaken feeling all right? Will he ask me questions that I don't want to answer? Will I be helpless?"

Not infrequently, patients harbor feelings that they don't express, i.e., "I wonder if he'll do to me what that cabaret hypnotist did when he stretched that person out like a board between two chairs, etc. I wonder if he'll make me do something I don't want to do. Will he put me under his power and transfer that power to others? I wonder if he could do me harm."

The fear of being hurt, victimized and being helpless can be very strong in some patients. Sometimes it is better to build warm rapport and confidence and to not proceed too rapidly in attempting to hypnotize a patient. It is very important to strongly emphasize that as a hypnotist you are only concerned with helping the patient to achieve what he desires, that both doctor and patient are pursuing the same aim. In this way the motivation of the patient consciously and subconsciously can be used to reinforce the patient's cooperation.

When the patient is exceptionally fearful, it is best not to rush with induction, but rather give the patient the feeling that you are in no hurry about it and that the patient should simply come and talk things over. Hypnotic induction is best attempted when the patient expresses a real desire to be hypnotized. With some anxious patients, pushing the matter of induction only heightens suspicions and fears, and can increase existing resistance.

If this approach is not taken, all too often the patient subconsciously brings old psychic defenses into play against "being made to do something that she doesn't really desire to do, i.e., this occurs frequently in patients seeking to be cured of their cigarette habit. Some are ambivalent, taking the position, "I don't want to quit smoking, but maybe he (the hypnotist) can make me quit."

But the "self" that has for years resisted giving up tobacco will not infrequently subconsciously balk and set up a defiance-resistance pattern against the treatment. This can manifest itself in all kinds of subtle attempts to sabotage the treatment.

Often when such patients recognize that they are at cross purposes with themselves, they can be persuaded to align themselves with the aims of the therapist. The latter must maintain steadfastly that he will only help the patient to achieve what he earnestly desires and will not engage in any battle of wills or resistance games.

Hypnosis is best presented to the patient, not as a suggestive technique, but preferably as a psychophysiological form of relaxation. This is more acceptable to most patients. They are less apt to see the doctor as some sort of Svengali or magician. The patient is told that he will not fall asleep but will enter into a wonderful twilight state between sleep and wakefulness which he will experience as very pleasant and relaxing. Further, that he will retain some awareness during the trance of his communications and his surroundings. He should be told that this psychophysiological relaxation (when possible the word "hypnosis" can be dispensed with) is beneficial to the physical and mental health, and that it has wonderful restorative effects, relieving fatigue tensions, making one feel refreshed, and greatly improving the subjective well being of the patient. In addition, the therapist should discuss with the patient his motives for seeking hypnosis, and carefully evaluate these. Patients who present no medically justifiable specific reason, indication or motivation, are generally speaking, not desirable subjects. However, there is an exception to this, and that is the patient who is generally unhappy, but who is unaware of the reasons for his difficulties and is actually in need of an exploration of his repressed conflicts and problems. This can be done effectively and rapidly in many cases under hypnosis, and this technique of hypnoanalysis has proved to be of considerable value. Once specific problems and conflicts have been uncovered, it is possible to plan a more specific program of hypnotherapy or psychotherapy for the patient.

It is often extremely difficult to evaluate the resistance of patients *a priori* because certain patients who subjectively give the impression of being cooperative are often quite resistive. Sometimes cooperation is feigned. On the other hand, there are patients who on the surface act very resistive but who can be easily relaxed into the hypnotic trance. Of considerable value in determining the susceptibility of the patient to hypnotic suggestion and induction is the handclasp test. (See Chapter four.) In the application of the Miller Induction Method, deep breathing in accordance with the initial test instructions indicate a marked conscious desire on the part of the patient to cooperate. Unconsciously motivated blocking, of course, may still occur. If this blocking or resistance is marked, the patient will not breathe deeply or, if so, only for a very brief period, or will breathe irregularly. He may try to speak or resist eye closure or continue voluntary movements, usually finger or arm movements or flicking of lids. If the patient is not resistive and is suggestive, he will continue to obey the instructions of the hypnotist during the induction process, going through stages of induction progressively. One must remember that patients often attempt during the initial phase to control the depth of their trance and therefore often give only limited cooperation. These patients are feeling their way, trying to gain reassurance, and should not be pressured too strongly. They should be told that they have responded splendidly and that with each successive induction they shall be able to respond better.

They should receive continued encouragement and as their anxiety lessens and they experience the beneficial effects of the hypnotic trance, they usually become better and better subjects. Since affectivity is greatly increased in the hypnotic state, it is, of course, possible to more readily recognize any marked anxiety reactions which the patients may present. Where there is marked anxiety or hysterical reactions, which persist, the trance should be promptly terminated. The reasons for this anxiety should be discussed. If manifested prior to the induction it should be discussed immediately; if manifested during the hypnotic trance, it should be explored during the trance and ventilated following the hypnotic trance. Since intellectual discriminatory functions are reduced in the hypnotic state and feelings are enhanced, it is best when questioning as to the source of their emotional disturbance to phrase the question as follows: "What is upsetting you more than anything else? or "What was the worst upset you've ever experienced as a child? etc. What was the worst thing that happened at home, in school, etc? What was the worst scare you ever had? Who upset you the most at home, in school, etc.?" The use of superlatives aids the patient in recalling the traumatic event. Recently a female patient, following a question of what upset her more than anything, "I needed to urinate and I didn't tell you. I was afraid I'd lose control of my bladder if I was hypnotized."

It is good to question resistive patients in the waking state or under hypnosis as follows: "Did you ever see anyone hypnotized? Did you ever see stage hypnosis? How did you feel when you saw them hypnotized, etc. Have you ever read about or discussed hypnosis with anyone? Do you have any feeling about people being hypnotized?" One male patient stated that he had been told by a minister of a particular sect that it was evil and the work of the devil.

Much can be done to arrive at the root of the conflict causing the anxiety or tension by means of hypnotic suggestion, suggesting in the trance that the patient shall desire in his own best interests to discuss the reasons for his anxiety and tension upon awakening. Reassurance, particularly in the initial phase, cannot be too strongly stressed, and is most important.

As discussed previously, it is most important *a priori* to explain the nature of the hypnotic state. Among other fears, there is often the fear of the unknown. This is important not only from the point of view of lessening the anxiety of the subject, but also to dispel the popular notion that one is unconscious, totally helpless, or unaware in the hypnotic trance. All too often patients otherwise will, on awakening from the trance, later remark that they hadn't felt they had been hypnotized because they knew what was said and they felt that they knew what was going on, they certainly could not have been hypnotized. The explanation that should be given before induction is that hypnosis is an altered and partially reduced state of consciousness between sleep and wakefulness, and that the patient may be acutely aware of specific sounds and remarks and his surroundings, in general, and that the degree of amnesia experienced may vary considerably in different individuals, depending on the depth of the trance. Posthypnotic amnesia can be usually induced by hypnotic suggestion.

Because a subject under hypnosis, especially during the first trance, is usually particularly wary of deception and of "being taken advantage of," it is best to proceed in such a way as to inspire his complete trust and faith. The more trust the subject feels, the more he will give in to and submit to the suggestions of the hypnotist. In subsequent sessions, the hypnotic influence can become very strong if such faith and trust exist, and this hypnotic influence can then be utilized in order to achieve marked therapeutic gains for the patient. During hypnosis, the patient can be greatly influenced by stressing factors which support his own personal desires and motivations. Trying to compel the subject to feel or act in opposition to his own inner motivation may not only create resistance and conflict, but may often bring the patient out of the hypnotic trance. Thus compelling the patient to act in opposition to his own inner wishes can seriously damage the therapeutic transference. It is always wise to put the patient's positive motivations to work for the hypnotist. Compelling him to act in a manner contrary to his real wishes may not only be harmful to the therapeutic process aforementioned, but may even result in marked anxiety and hysterical symptom formation. Patients will generally unconsciously create defenses against the threat which they feel, and usually become increasingly resistive. One must never lose sight of the high degree of sensitivity and vulnerability of the hypnotized patient. It is necessary to make him feel secure and unthreatened, to build positive rapport and trust.

The motivations of the patient for submitting to hypnosis may be manifold. There may be a desire to find relief from symptoms, painful pressures, tensions and pain or to seek some magical solutions to a problem. In some there may exist a desire to escape from painful reality. Often, patients who are literally desperate for help seek hypnotherapy as a sort of last resort since other types of treatment had failed to help them. Sometimes a person cannot consciously face his conflicts and seeks hypnotherapy out of desperation as a less painful alternative to facing the dreaded encounter in the waking state. Often a patient who is in a highly tense state may readily submit to hypnosis because it affords the possibility of either help or an escape. The reasons or motives for the escape desire should be carefully explored. The desire as aforementioned for a magical cure often represents a regressive childlike wish on the part of the patient. There are many persons, for instance, who rather than struggle with frequent repetitive desires for food or cigarettes would much prefer, if possible, having an unconscious aversion to these created in them by hypnosis so that the continuous conflict is eliminated. Quite frequently, patients will use the motive of "I want to quit smoking or overeating" or some other bad habit as a pretext to seeking psychotherapeutic aid, and will later admit this as their real need. Certainly, it is also most important to utilize the hypnotic session to attempt to uncover the emotional starvation, frustration and conflicts which are almost always at the root of the compulsive eating, smoking, or drinking. We all seek to avoid pain, tension and anguish, and to attain pleasure and mental peace. Hypnosis provides a ready psychic escape into a pleasurable and peaceful state of mind. The marked desire of patients to experience this peaceful and tranquil state of mind is often manifest in the fact that many hypnotic subjects linger before emerging from their trance. It is understandable that the tense patient frequently may seek to prolong the peaceful and relaxed state of mind. The underlying reasons should be explored, whenever possible, as to why the patient is so strongly resisting returning to the reality situation. What does reality present that is so disturbing or painful? There are those patients who seek at least temporarily to regress back to an infantile—oral level, such as for example, alcoholics, drug addicts, etc., the nirvana and peaceful bliss, the submission to an all-powerful and strong parental figure, namely the hypnotist. It is, of course, impossible to set up a standard formula for all persons who submit to hypnosis, anymore than it is possible to set up a similar standard for alcoholics. There are many causes for human suffering, dependency, and ego weakness, and they must be explored in the individual patient. Similarly, there are as many causes, for example, for alcoholism, as there are for human unhappiness and pain.

As stated previously, when inducing hypnosis, the author has found that patients submit much more rapidly if they anticipate a very pleasurable state of relaxation from an existing state of tension. Who doesn't want to feel better? Hypnosis can provide a ready release for pent-up, disturbing emotions. Usually, the patient will ventilate these in the hypnotic trance and if the patient is sufficiently rational and not too disturbed, the conflicts can be later consciously reviewed with the patient. This conscious ventilation of problems not only helps to relieve tension, to further the insight of the patient, but also is an ego strengthening device in that it teaches the patient that he can face problems without breaking down.

While under hypnosis, not only the central motivations in the patient's life, such as pleasure, success, happiness and good health, but also his real problems should not be obscured. He should be helped to become aware of the real causes of his difficulties and what possible solutions there are. He should be given added ego strength to solve these problems; he should not be removed from the world situation but confronted with it; to the extent that he is able to cope, and that when he has initial success in solving these problems, he will gain added ego strength and continue to make therapeutic gains. In this way he does not become helplessly dependent on the therapist.

The hypnotist should, if possible, always remain with his patient. If he leaves the patient, the patient's anxiety may be intensified and he may emerge from the trance. If the hypnotist must leave for a brief period, he should reassure the patient, telling him that he will soon return and to remain comfortable and relaxed, and enjoy his very pleasant relaxation, in fact, that when he returns the patient will be even more deeply relaxed. If indicated, he can engage the patient in counting, breathing, or hand levitation, or some sort of trance-deepening process during the time he is absent from the patient. Or he can resort to preoccupying the patient with attempts to recall significant past memories, events and material relevant to his present concerns.

There are many misconceptions about hypnosis; there are many unnecessary anxieties. One only has to reflect on the original committee of great scientists who investigated Mesmer's work and who were apparently so affected by all the prevailing professional bias against Mesmer at the time, they did not objectively review the great number of patients who had experienced real benefits from his treatment.

Many of the misconceptions regarding hypnosis have, unfortunately, been the result of the use of hypnosis by untrained persons and quacks, and also because of exaggerated claims. Hypnosis can be a valuable and potent instrument for helping human beings; for diagnosis and treatment. But, like surgery, it must be left in the hands of well-trained professional experts. Because of the atmosphere out of which hypnosis has emerged, out of mysticism and magic, out of pseudoscientific and the circus sideshow, it is to be anticipated that lay persons generally would feel uneasy and anxious about undergoing hypnosis. There are such fears as "I don't want to be dominated by the will of another," or "I don't want to lose control over myself," or "What will happen to me if I give up control over myself or my mind to some sort of Svengali?" or "All this seems strange and unnatural to me." Of course, the doctor must explain that it is a method which requires both the cooperation of the doctor and the patient, is positively nonharmful, and in fact, the relaxation is beneficial; he must give reassurance and support in order to overcome the patient's anxieties. In cases in which the anxiety of the patient is such that he cannot cooperate, we have found it useful at our clinic to tell patients that we would like to test their capacity for relaxation. This testing procedure has been so efficacious that I now use it as a standard procedure. They are then put through a combination of the endogenic procedure of breathing exercises (see Chapter four), and are soon relaxed into the initial trance. After the initial trance, the patient will emerge relaxed, often slightly drowsy, generally feeling very much relieved and in an excellent frame of mind, and thereafter the procedure is a very simple one.

Considerations on Initial Induction

It is important that the patient prior to the hypnotic induction is not proccupied with any disturbing problem which may distract his interest, attention and concentration. Concern or anxiety over an appointment, a child returning from school, or something that had not been taken care of on the job, or duty or errand, or simply a mundane matter such as relieving the bladder or rectum, may affect the patient's capacity to relax into the hypnotic state. This is primarily because any preoccupation, anxiety or tension of this kind may seriously interfere with the capacity of the patient to concentrate. Concentration is of the utmost importance in hypnotic induction. Concentration as well as rapport and the suggestibility of the patient are the three principal psychic factors in the induction process. Concentration is heightened by a feeling of trust and security. Each is dependent on the other, so that patients who have good rapport with the hypnotist are able to concentrate much better and show a higher degree of suggestibility. Marked concentration aids and facilitates the disassociative process and the reality withdrawal which occurs progressively during hypnotic induction. It is, of course, a clinical fact that patients who are ill are often narcissistically preoccupied with their own illness and symptoms, their body, their health and life security. They are primarily preoccupied with the problem of getting relief for their suffering and attempting to gain security by resolving their fears of sickness and death. This fact can be successfully exploited by the therapist in a sympathetic approach to their problem, and attempting to ally himself with the patient's pursuit of assistance and relief from his suffering and illness. Any attempt at this point to divert the patient from his self-preoccupation towards an external object, such as may be done in certain forms of hypnotic induction involving the utilization of external fixations or stimulations, may be reacted to in a negative manner by the patient. Moreover, it is generally difficult for a patient in this state to externalize and fixate his attention easily. It has been our experience that when the concentration is focused on a bodily function of the patient such as respiration, as is done in the endogenic method, the patient tends to cooperate to a fuller degree and is able to better concentrate and achieve a higher degree of suggestibility more rapidly. Concentration on his own bodily function, in this instance respiration, is facilitated by eye closure, and by repeated, modulated instructions to the patient to carefully observe his respiratory rhythm, inspiration and expiration, and the rate of breathing, and to carefully watch for the test changes in the respiratory rhythm which he shall, as a result of the instructions, come to anticipate.

The concentration process can, of course, be disturbed by numerous factors. Foremost among these are such emotional tensions as anxiety, anger, frustration or

tensions resulting from interference, delay, insecurity, un-
fulfilled duties or responsibilities, etc. Other disturbing factors to the patient can be excessive noise, light or moving
objects. The treatment environment should be conducive
to concentration just as the bedroom is conducive to rest
and sleep. For this purpose, a comfortable couch is best,
with a comfortable head rest or cushion. I prefer to use a
recliner which can be adjusted to the patient's comfort. The
patient must above all feel comfortable and the hypnotist
should be very solicitous in his manner toward the patient,
sympathetically regarding his feelings and state of comfort.
It is very important to consider the initial anxieties that a
patient feels when first confronting treatment by hypnosis.
The patient, being unaware of what it means to be hypnotized, reflects the usual fears of the unknown, "Well, I don't
know what it will be like . . ." in an anxious voice. It should
be patiently and gently explained to the patient that hypnosis represents an altered state of consciousness during
which he will feel wonderfully relaxed, and that the peaceful relaxation is not only very beneficial to the mind, but
relaxing to the heart and the entire body. Further, he
should be told that he will remain in contact with reality
and aware of what is going on. It is further explained that
he can be readily awakened when the treatment is finished,
and that upon awakening he will feel very comfortable and
relaxed. Many patients are somewhat disturbed and anxious that the treatment might upset them in some way, and
they must be reassured on this point. Furthermore, it must
be carefully explained to him that being hypnotized does
not mean a complete loss of consciousness, since many
patients will complain afterwards that they have not been
hypnotized because they have not lost their awareness of
their surroundings. It should be further explained that the
success of the treatment depends in large measure on the
cooperation of the patient and his earnest desire for help.
Patients are told that if they feel like that, they'll have no

difficulty passing the induction test. Such an explanation helps to protect the therapist from blame if the induction or treatment is unsuccessful. It is the patient who has failed the test. Furthermore, it suggests in the event of failure, that if the patient is more cooperative, further treatment can be successful, and he will be able to pass the test soon. Concentration during the induction procedure can be intensified by a number of devices. Primary among these is counting. Counting backward, such as counting from 20 to one tends to effect greater concentration than counting forward. Other concentration devices are, for example, hand levitation, or as aforementioned, concentrating on the respiratory rhythm or the depth, and sensory and motor changes. Furthermore, as previously noted, concentration can be enhanced by developing a keen sense of anticipation in the patient that gradually changes will occur, such as, for example, the change in respiratory rhythm, in skin sensation, in muscular relaxation, or change in the state of psychic relaxation, etc. With reference to hand levitation, the patient's attention can be called to the changes he will feel in his hand, that his hand will become increasingly light; that he will first feel movement in certain fingers, and that then this feeling of movement and lightness will spread from the fingers to the hand and then to the arm, etc.

Of considerable importance, too, is the hypnotist's voice. Instructions to the patient should be given in a measured, kindly, regular, fairly monotone, but authoritative voice, suggesting rest and relaxation, and in such a manner so as not to disturb the concentration process. Rather the intent should be to enhance the concentration by constantly stressing the observation or focusing of attention on the breathing of the patient or on the sensation of lightness and elevation in the case of hand levitation. Concentration can also be intensified by utilizing positive purposeful motivation, as for example, the need to obtain relief from suffering, and the pleasures, joys, and successes that will follow the treatment. In this connection it should be pointed out that the patient cooperates best when he desires to find relief from his sufferings, which in many cases, may be unbearable. It is good, in the initial interview, to allow the patient to elaborate on his symptoms and suffering and to listen sympathetically. Furthermore, it is good to respond optimistically if the treatment outlook can be favorable. Fostering a positive anticipatory sense that he will achieve relief generally tends to markedly accentuate concentration and motivation. As previously noted, favorable rapport greatly facilitates concentration. The patient can always more readily externalize his concentrated interest on an object, in this instance, the hypnotist, if he reacts to him in a positive manner. Thus the personality of the hypnotist assumes great importance. The withdrawal of interest by a subject from other persons is indicative of resistance toward them. As noted previously, the proper exploitation of the anticipation mechanism can be a very important factor in facilitating concentration. In this regard, suggestive influences, i.e., prestige, reputation of hypnotist, particularly if they prevail in the mind of the patient prior to the induction of the hypnotic trance, may greatly facilitate concentration.

In his preliminary interview with the patient, the hypnotist should determine what influences preexist in the patient's mind, so that he can stimulate these later by means of hypnotic suggestion. The hypnotist must learn to exploit every positive factor to the advantage of the therapeutic process. The patient is often eagerly awaiting his experience with the hypnotist and the effects upon himself. It is this conception of the hypnosis and the effects upon himself which, if possible, should be obtained from the patient prior to induction. Repeated suggestion is used, of course, to strengthen the patient's concentration. Where previous inductions have occurred, concentration can be intensified by means of posthypnotic suggestion. In such cases, the patient is spontaneously obeying an unconscious command. This influence when sufficiently reinforced by strong verbal repetition, can represent a powerful motivating force in some instances.

There are additional factors which affect the concentration and induction process, such as (1) the *trust* which the patient feels in the therapist; (2) the *realization* that the trance is only for the purpose of fulfilling the purposes and life objectives which the patient so much desires; (3) that the patient fully understands the nature of the procedure and is fully in accord with the objectives to be pursued; (4) that the patient is sufficiently free of anxiety and sufficiently comprehends the likely benefits of the hypnosis procedure as regards his health and happiness; (6) the aforementioned rapport factors play an important role in creating positive transference feelings towards the therapist, making the patient much more susceptible to hypnotic induction and treatment.

Already James Braid correctly believed that it was not so much the visual fixation of the subject but the concentration of his attention that was the significant factor in the hypnotic induction. On the other hand, Bernheim believed that suggestion was the key to all hypnotic phenomena, while Sidis stressed the importance of rapport. There is no doubt that all of these are basic requisites, and that they reinforce each other. In the opinion of the author, the hypnotic induction is achieved primarily through the psychic concentration on a fixed stimuli in addition to relaxation suggestion, as in the case of endogenic induction, for example, on the respiratory function, the subsequent changes. Self-observation heightens concentration. Weitzenhoffer has pointed out that the prior conviction, if established, that sensory fixation brings about hypnosis tends in itself to act as a suggestion and the phenomena results. He goes on to point out that the concentrated attention does not appear to be a precondition for all trance inductions. No doubt this often occurs; however, this is certainly manifest in later repeated inductions (dressage phenomenon).

What of the suggestions that the patient is becoming fatigued? Are such suggestions, such as eye closure is occurring, necessary? In the opinion of the author, no. With the endogenic method all of this is for the most part obsolete. Eye closure is practiced from the very onset. It is explained to the patient that this is done as a preventive measure, to prevent drying and irritation of the cornea of the eye and unnecessary eye strain. Whatever is told, the subject must make sense in terms of the reality to him. Fatiguing the patient generally results in frustration, tension and the development of resistance. Hence, it generally impairs rather than facilitates therapeutic transference. There are cases of resistance to hypnotic induction in which suggestive techniques of an indirect type have often been found to be effective in what may be otherwise highly refractory patients. As indicated earlier, lapses of attention and concentration, or the subject trying to divert his attention from the hypnotist is generally a manifestation of resistance and needs to be promptly discussed and ventilated. In this connection, eavesdropping, the use of the auxiliary hypnotist, muscle relaxation, dermal touch—pain desensitization, etc. may be very useful.

Chapter 4

HYPNOTIC INDUCTION

Since first reported by James Braid in 1843, various external fixation methods have been employed for the purpose of hypnotic induction. Liebeault combined the Braid method with suggestion. Autorelaxation methods were practiced in a modified degree for centuries by the Yogiists who utilized breathing relaxation and mind over body control procedures, teaching their disciples breathing and muscle control among other methods as a conscious disciplinary exercise. In more recent years J. Schultz applied stage-by-stage hypnotic relaxation with his so-called autogenic training methods in which he would train subjects in psychosomatic relaxation of various body parts by a progressive step-by-step procedure.

THE BRAID-LIEBEAULT PROCEDURE

In the Braid-Liebeault procedure the patient is instructed to fixate on a point or an object in the room. Some have used moving objects as well. Peripheral light should best be dimmed so that fixation on a specific point is facilitated. The patient is told that his eyelids are becoming heavier and heavier and he is relaxing deeper and deeper. As he relaxes deeper and deeper his eyelids are closing as he falls into deeper and deeper hypnotic relaxation. After eye closure is achieved, the trance can be deepened by hand levitation.

In view of the fact that I, like many of my colleagues, have consistently encountered certain difficulties with standard fixation and progressive relaxation methods of hypnotic induction, I was prompted to explore the possibilities of a more practical and effective procedure. In my experience, the principal difficulties with the previously mentioned standard methods are:

1. The length of time usually required for induction;
2. The resistance thus created in the subject as well as resistance to fixation procedures per se;
3. The consequent higher percent of failures in induction;
4. The great effort required by the hypnotist and the subject;
5. The difficulties encountered whenever attempting to utilize such methods for purposes of demonstrating to students and colleagues, etc.

After employing other procedures for hypnotic induction, i.e., the classical Braid procedure, metronome, the Schultz autogenic training method, the hand-levitation method, and others, I discovered that there were disadvantages to all of these methods. All of these procedures generally required more time than my endogenic method. Secondly, they (particularly the Braid method) involved optic fixation plus relaxation suggestion; often they proved wearing on both the patient and the hypnotist. The endogenic method was far more effective than the Braid and similar methods depending on repetitive sensory stimulation plus relaxation suggestion. Schultz's method was effective and in particular, useful, for trance deepening but because of the time involved, I found it rather impractical for clinical use when time was a factor. It was particularly time-consuming on initial inductions.

For trance deepening, the procedure I utilize is as follows: The patient's arm is lifted and it is suggested that it is very heavy and it is getting heavier and heavier and will fall like a dead weight and as it falls, the patient will fall off deeper into the trance. After the arm is down, the patient is told that a helium balloon is being attached to his wrist which will lift his arm up to make a delightful contact with the forehead. After the fingers of the hypnotist encircle the wrist of the patient to attach the helium balloon effect, the wrist is drawn slightly upward as the hypnotist's fingers disengage with the accompanying suggestion that the hand and arm are elevating. This usually tends to facilitate and speed up hand levitation. It is suggested that the higher the arm goes, the more delightful and relaxed the patient will feel. When contact is made with his forehead, he is told that he will receive a deep hypnotic transfusion through his brain and body and become so limp and relaxed all over that his arm would drop like a dead weight. After his arm drops, it is placed in a comfortable position and he is told that he will fall off even deeper.

SUSCEPTIBILITY TESTS

Susceptibility tests precede induction. I only use susceptibility tests when indicated. Usually the routine respiratory three-stage test procedure is sufficient. See endogenic method, p. 80. If the patient appears refractory, susceptibility tests can be employed.

There are a considerable variety of susceptibility tests. I have found the following tests helpful.

1. The patient is turned and given a suggestion that he is falling backwards. The therapist stands behind the patient so that he can feel secure and fall back safely.

2. Have the patient stretch out his hands and instruct him to keep them parallel at the same level in front of him. Then instruct him to close his eyes and to maintain his hands at the same level, while suggesting that one arm is drifting downward or laterally.

3. Have the patient close his eyes and breathe deeply suggesting that his breathing is getting shallower. Observe his compliance.

4. Feel the patient's pulse and respiration and suggest that his pulse or respiration is speeding or slowing up. Observe the changes, if any.

5. Hand clasp test. This test originated with the famous French autosuggestionist, Emile Coue. The patient stands facing the therapist, arms outstretched rigidly and hands clasped together, fingers intertwined. In a commanding manner the suggestion is given that the tighter the patient squeezes his hands together, the more they become locked together—so tightly the patient cannot open them, even on command ("on the count of three") of the therapist.

Always, always tell the patient that you are going to test his susceptibility to undergoing hypnotic induction and that as soon as he succeeds in the initial phase of testing, you will put him deeper, thereby testing his capacity to go into a deeper and deeper trance. If the patient fails to achieve the hypnotic state, he will feel that he hasn't passed the test rather than blaming the hypnotist and accusing him of incompetence. This is very important because then the hypnotist has not lost the patient's trust and can maintain his prestige and authority in the eyes of the patient. There-fore, he is better able to attempt a subsequent induction. He can then first discuss and try to resolve the causes of resistance, i.e., anxiety, subconscious defiance, embarrassment, curiosity, etc. Banal factors such as worrying about being late to work or for an appointment or a need to go to the toilet can markedly interfere with induction. Physical factors such as noise, bright light, excessive cold or heat, an irritable secretary or receptionist, can greatly disturb the induction process. Check whether the patient is wearing contact lenses. Many who do, find eye-closure uncomfortable. Lack of warmth, tension or signs of impatience or irritability on the part of the hypnotist are marked deterrents. Assurances of complete privacy and quiet are highly essential.

RAPPORT

Establishing good rapport is essential. Some of the major determinants of rapport in hypnosis are:

1. Personality rapport depends very much on personality interreaction, i.e., aggressive, dominant females may feel less threatened by a more passive, reserved hypnotist. If the hypnotist impresses as dominant and authoritative, it may set off a defiance resistance contest—a reliving of earlier patterns with such a patient. If the patient is a more dependent, nonassertive type, then he may feel more secure toward a strong, authoritative parent figure as the hypnotist.

2. It is important to greet the patient warmly, in a relaxed manner. (A warm, accepting receptionist helps rapport as does the initial warmth and cordiality of the hypnotist. For example, while a patient is waiting to be seen, the receptionist may offer him a cup of tea or coffee.)

3. Getting a careful, unhurried history of the patient is also important. Let him discuss his conception of hypnosis. Clear up and resolve any misconceptions he might have. Take time to explain what hypnosis is like, that it is merely an altered state of consciousness, a partial sleep state, a very delightful, pleasant, relaxed state which creates increased feelings of euphoria (well-being) and comfort.

Explain that the patient is not helpless and is essentially aware of what is going on, that he is not asleep and his hearing may even become sharper. After the initial explanation, allow the patient to express his anticipatory feelings about being hypnotized. Fears of loss of control should be resolved. Some patients express fears of "How will I awaken from the trance? Can any harmful effects occur?" These anxieties should be allayed. Motivation to submitting to hypnosis is greatly enhanced by warm rapport, by a feeling of trust.

4. A personal interest shown by the hypnotist can greatly increase rapport with suggestions to the patient that, if he has some habit or inclination which disturbs or troubles him, he might mention it and the hypnotist will try to help him overcome it, e.g., getting up late, not concentrating on his studies, etc. Frequently it helps induction rapport and motivation greatly to have patients write up a list of problems, habits, or inhibitions that they would like to understand, get rid of or change. It is very important for rapport to make the patient feel that the hypnotist only desires to fulfill the wishes of the patient, to only help him achieve his desires, and not to compel him in any way.

5. Where it is possible, a major factor in rapport is the recommendation from patients successfully treated. That is to say, rapport is rapidly or in part already established if the patient was referred by a satisfied former patient, or else if one patient successfully treated is introduced to a new patient in the waiting room.

In cases where the patient resists initial induction, and after insight and rapport are achieved and resistance largely resolved, a second attempt to induce hypnosis can be made, i.e., "I will now test you again. I am sure that everything will go much better for you." Then the hypnotist can proceed with the test and the induction usually without much difficulty. Sometimes some idea of the patient's state of mind is gotten by a simple question: "Would you like to attempt the test again?" If there is doubt or hesitancy expressed, it would be best to defer the attempt to another occasion when the patient is desiring the treatment.

As previously mentioned, a popular and commonly used procedure for induction is the hand levitation method. The patient should be told to close his eyes to avoid drying of the eyes which causes irritation. One hand is dropped alongside of the chair and he is given repeated suggestions that his hand is getting lighter and lighter, so light that it will rise upward. Suggestions are given that it is rising higher and higher, that it will continue to rise higher and faster until it makes contact with the forehead. When it reaches the forehead, give suggestions that a hypnotic transfusion is occurring which will relax the patient into a deeper and deeper hypnotic trance and that as he goes deeper, he will be more and more relaxed and better and better.

I favor my own endogenic method because it is more reliable and generally more rapid and involves a psychophysiological approach. Furthermore, it is considerably more effective particularly with resistive patients and especially with those who resent Svengali methods.

Passes have been used by some hypnotists on selected subjects. This relies to a large extent on the patient's degree of suggestibility and susceptibility to magical effects and the faith and awe for the authority and power of the hypnotist. The visual attention of the subject is caught and the hand of the hypnotist is passed before the eyes of the subject, as hypnotic relaxation is suggested. A touch on the forehead plus suggestion can enhance the effect. In my experience, I have found that the pass is more useful as a posthypnotic induction technique. While under hypnosis, the subject is told that a pass between his eyes or a touch to his forehead will put him into a spontaneous trance.

THE MILLER ENDOGENIC METHOD*

I have chosen the term "endogenic" as a means of distinguishing my procedure from past methods which were largely based on external fixation, on a respiratory cerebral reflex, the Hering-Breuer phenomenon, which regulates the breathing depth and frequency due to changes in the carbon dioxide-oxygen ratio in the blood stream. In the endogenic technique, concentration is on the subject's own respiratory rhythm and external influence is reduced to a minimum. (Note chain reaction of suggestion.)

With the revival of the use of hypnosis on a larger scale for clinical purposes, it appeared imperative that an attempt be made to develop a more suitable clinical procedure. Many colleagues had objected to the use of hypnosis on the grounds that it was entirely too time-consuming and often unpredictable and unreliable. There have been some attempts to relax patients by respiratory means, i.e., the work done by Sargent and Fraser who experimented with forced breathing and hyperventilation but who did not employ hypnotic suggestion at all. Their efforts were apparently discontinued due to the fact that prolonged hyper-

*The endogenic method was first demonstrated by the author at the Wagner-Juaregg Clinic, Vienna, and at the International Conference on Psychotherapy, Barcelona, Spain in 1958.

ventilation resulted in a disturbance of acid-base balance and a consequent state of alkalotic tetany. Further Leitner and Weitzenhoffer pointed to the observation that deep inspiration heightened the suggestibility of patients. Already the ancient Talmudists were aware of the relaxation produced by free expansive breathing and the fact that constricted breathing was associated with fear.

I found in my research that a continuous external stimulus seemed not only to fatigue and frustrate but in some cases to divert the subject's attention from relaxation; consequently increasing resistance so well paraphrased in a patient's remark, "I am so tired of looking at that damn pen." I noted further that withdrawal from the outer world was facilitated by concentration upon the subject's own self. Every form of suggestion represents to a degree an attempt to outwit the subject's ego. I agree entirely with Erickson and Wolberg that the hypnotist should ally himself with the patient's will and objectives rather than against them. I felt further that if the subject was given a real indication of the hypnotist's knowledge and capacity to predict his reactions, the subject would be thus rendered more suggestible and amenable to hypnotic relaxation. I thus decided, after a number of preliminary experiments to employ the following method.

(Note: Induction is done with the patient in the reclining position. Again, contact lenses should be removed.)

The subject was told to close his eyes, "First, you will close your eyelids and keep them closed until I instruct you to reopen them." It was explained that, in this manner, excessive eye strain, drying of the eyes and irritation can be avoided. I found that generally eye closure facilitated concentration of self and one's own bodily functions. If the patient wishes, the mechanism of induction is first explained briefly to the patient. He is told (1) that slow, deep respiration will cause an oxygen overload in the bloodstream; (2) that this overload will affect the respiratory center in the medulla, causing a marked change in his breathing rhythm with a slowing of the heart and respiration, relaxing the entire mind and body progressively; (3) that this effect will spread quite rapidly from the hind brain over the mid and fore brain, inducing a very pleasant progressive relaxation of mind and body; and (4) that he will feel drowsy and sleepy but at no time will he lose contact with the therapist. He will be able to hear the therapist's voice and to express himself freely and without effort.

The author attempts to exploit the Hering-Breuer respiratory reflex in this manner. This phenomenon results from stimulation of the pulmonary fibers of the Vagus, thus automatically inhibiting and regulating respiration. The patient is made to strongly anticipate these effects. The subject is instructed further that he must carefully observe and concentrate on the character of his breathing and its rhythm and that this will be an exact indicator of the degree of his relaxation. It is very necessary to engage the patient's ego in intense concentration on his respiratory function, since I have found that subjects are far more suggestible when under intense concentration. This is because the ego is so engaged that it cannot resist suggestion as effectively. Furthermore, the psyche becomes more suggestible progressively as the induction progresses. Under no circumstances is the patient permitted to force-breathe. He is instructed to breathe slowly, deeply and rhythmically. Generally, I do not wait for an actual change in the respiratory rhythm but suggest that this change is already perceptible and that relaxation now will rapidly follow. The subject is then further told that his respiration is markedly changing and that he is responding splendidly just as he should. It should be repeated a number of times in a continually more modulated and gentle voice that the relaxation is going to be increasingly more pleasant, and that tensions and concerns will rapidly dissipate. (Note: The process of hypnotic relaxation can often be speeded up by the utilization of the author's technique of employing an auxiliary hypnotist.)

A step-by-step description of the actual induction procedure employed in the Miller Endogenic Method is as follows:

Phase one:

Tell the patient, "Breathe deeply and slowly." Watch for three test signs which will now occur as the patient relaxes:

1. "Your chest breathing will change to belly breathing."
2. "Your belly breathing will become shallower and level off."
3. "Your toes will deviate" (either outwardly or inwardly depending on whether they are together or apart.) (If done in the sitting position, the third test sign given is to the effect that the head will fall forward, back or sideways depending on which way the head is inclining.)

Phase two:

1. Tell the patient, "Since you have passed the first test, I am going to take you deeper. You will now breathe deeply again."
2. "You will feel a beautiful tranquil feeling going all through you, through your mind and body."
3. "You will feel a delightful sense of well-being and comfort" (euphoria).
4. "You will feel a progressively deeper feeling of drowsiness."
5. "Soon your breathing will become virtually imperceptible as you are experiencing progressively deeper muscle relaxation."

Phase three:

1. Continue telling the patient, "You are relaxing so well that I'm going to take you to a deeper level by means of the 'count' which is a deepening procedure."
2. "I will now count down from 30 to one. Each count will take you deeper. When I reach one, you will be deeply relaxed.
3. The count begins 30 to 19. "At 19, I'm reversing the count so you can go even deeper." Count to 29 and then to the subject: "Now the double reversal and you will go doubly deep with every count as I count down to one. When I reach one, you will be very deeply relaxed."

Phase four:

"I will now test your trance depth by lifting your left leg. It is very limp and heavy (hypotonic). As I drop it, you are falling off more deeply. I will now test your right leg and as I raise and drop it, you will fall off even deeper. I will now test your right arm and as I lift and drop it, you will fall off deeper yet. As I test your left arm and drop it into the deep hypnotic void, you will fall off even deeper." The arm is dropped into the empty space alongside couch or chair.

Phase five: Hand levitation.

"I'm now attaching a helium balloon effect to your left wrist." (This can be done by grasping the patient's wrist for a moment and giving it a slight lift upward as the hypnotist's hand disengages.) "You will feel an increasingly strong pull upward as your left hand gets lighter and lighter. Your hand is moving upwardly. Soon it will go into the 'sweep' like the sweep of the second hand of a fine watch continuing nonstop to the forehead. As the hand rises, you are going deeper and deeper into the beautiful hypnotic relaxation."

Challenge—As the hand elevates, the patient is commanded to open his eyes and observe the hand elevating under hypnotic power. "You now realize you are hypnotized and go even further into deep hypnotic relaxation." Then he is told, "Your eyes will now close tightly as you relax into a very deep hypnotic sleep."

"Now you will make contact with your forehead and as you do, you will experience a beautiful, deep transfusion of hypnotic trance effect all through your brain and body until you become so relaxed that your hand falls limply downward. As it does, you will fall off even deeper." After it drops, then the hand is placed by the hypnotist in a comfortable position. "As I place your hand in a comfortable position, you fall off even deeper. You will take my voice and instructions with you at all times. Whatever I convey to you will be indelibly impressed on your mind and you will carry out my instructions for your benefit. Each time I instruct you to relax in the future, you will be able to relax more deeply and more rapidly into an even more pleasant and deep hypnotic trance."

TESTING RELAXATION AND TRANCE DEPTH

The degree of the relaxation of the patient can now be tested by: (1) testing muscle tone. If the patient is under deeply, muscle tone will be greatly reduced, the muscles rather flaccid. The tendon reflexes may remain and are often found hyperactive; (2) If very deeply relaxed catalepsy (trance-like state may occur in which voluntary motion is lost and a peculiar plastic rigidity of the muscles occurs by reason of which, i.e., the hand tends to retain for an indefinite time any position in which it is placed); (3) by hand levitation method (subjective feeling of lightness and raising of arm occurs upon suggestion); (4) by testing compliance with commands; (5) affectivity response, by suggesting the patient will feel temporary tingling or numbness in a specific area, "Somatic suggestibility"; (7) by the pain-stimulus response. If the patient is under deeply, he will perceive little or no cutaneous pain sensation, if it is strongly suggested to him preferably several times that he will feel no pain; (8) posthypnotic suggestion. The latter procedure is excellent in order to evaluate the degree of therapeutic influence which the therapist has exercised over the patient. For instance, patients being treated for the first time for nicotinism are told that their first act on awakening would be to forget their cigarettes in my office before they left. Upon awakening they most promptly complied. This act, in my opinion, was a very good prognostic indication regarding abstinence from cigarettes and the strength of the posthypnotic suggestion.

When the hypnotic session is completed, the patient is told, "I will count out silently until 20 and the last ten count outloud. At the count of 30, you will awaken feeling very refreshed and wonderful." Upon awakening, the subject may yawn, stretch, rub his eyes as though awakening from a deep sleep. If the patient has simulated induction and is resisting, he will probably not answer when questioned and when repeatedly commanded to respond may open his eyes. Prompt response and cooperation of the subject are good indicators of a satisfactory induction.

TRANCE DEEPENING TECHNIQUES

This can be accomplished by repeatedly lifting the extremities, suggesting greater limpness and deepening hypnotic relaxation, or, in addition, by suggesting that each time the hypnotist touches the patient's forehead he will go deeper. When using the visual induction method (Braid) passes can be used, i.e., passing the hand between the eyes, suggesting deepening relaxation. Thus, by means of progressive relaxation and repetitive pyramiding of suggestion, the trance can be deepened.

Trance deepening can also be accomplished by giving sleep relaxation suggestion while compressing the temples. Another compression point that can be used is the cervical spine at the base of the occipital area. An effective deepening procedure is circumduction of the arm. The extended arm is taken by the hypnotist in a circular motion, giving suggestions that the subject is going deeper and deeper. The suggestion is given that the arm is getting heavier and heavier and is guided by the wrist lower and lower until it makes contact with the patient's chest and the subject is told that it will then come to rest as he goes ever deeper.

Trance depth can be increased by any one or a combination of the following techniques.

1. Slowing and lengthening the count, i.e., from 30 to 40. If great depth is desired, the count can also be lengthened by counting down from 50–100. Reverse counting is an excellent deepening procedure. The hypnotist counts until the verge of awakening, i.e., to 39 instead of 40 and then reverses, suggesting that the patient will go very deep with every count downward until one.
2. Taking the patient into a trance several days in a row, suggesting that he will go progressively deeper every time he goes under. (Phenomenon of dressage.)
3. Challenging the patient as he lifts his hand toward forehead, telling him to open his eyes and observe the hand rising under hypnotic power. This usually convinces him that he is hypnotized. He is then told that he will now close his eyes and go into a very deep trance.

4. Instructing patients that as they go deeper, the count down will be speeded up. (This also requires less time.)
5. Giving the suggestion that every time their leg or arm is dropped, they will go progressively deeper.
6. Instructing them that when they breathe more deeply again, each breath will take them deeper into the trance until they have reached a very deep level. They will then note that their breathing has become very still.

Deepening of the trance can also be achieved by my method of employing an observer, a nurse, receptionist or colleague as an auxiliary hypnotist. (See p. 91.)

Indications of increased trance depth are:

1. Marked immobility
2. Shallow respiration
3. Hypotonia marked
4. Catalepsy may be marked
5. Highly suggestible
6. Very compliant
7. Capacity to regress marked
8. Posthypnotic suggestibility markedly increased, i.e., the patient is given the suggestion that after awakening he will leave his cigarettes on my desk and forget that he laid them there. Further, the suggestion is given that on awakening he will count quickly to ten but leave out the number nine. When the patient awakens simply repeat the instruction. "Count from one to ten."

I also employ the following procedures to facilitate reinduction.

After the patient has been inducted one or more times and is responding well, posthypnotic suggestion can be employed to the effect that if the hypnotist counts down from ten or five to one, the subject will promptly go into a deep trance. The post-hypnotic suggestion is continually reinforced that "Each time I instruct you to relax, you will go progressively deeper and faster into the trance." Post-hypnotic suggestions can be given that "Each time I touch you on the forehead or on the left shoulder you will go even deeper." Posthypnotic suggestion can be made that "When I (the hypnotist) pass my hand across your eyes or downward between your eyes, you will follow my hand and fall off into a deep trance."

TRANCE PROLONGATION TECHNIQUE

When a patient is under hypnosis, the unconscious ego, depending upon inner motivation, struggles to either prolong the trance or reattain the conscious wakeful state, and sooner or later the patient will emerge from his trance. It was apparent that it was necessary to utilize the influence of the unconscious ego as a therapeutic device rather than to permit it to thwart the therapeutic objective. At this point, the pleasure principle of Freud which plays such a powerful role in unconsciously motivating human reactions was applied. The patients were told under hypnosis that if they permitted themselves to emerge from their sleep relaxation, they would suffer disagreeable restlessness and discomfort. But, on the other hand, if they kept themselves in painless sleep relaxation until the hypnotist gives specific instructions for awakening, they would enjoy a continuous, pleasurable, restful, wonderful sleep from which they would awaken refreshed and rested, with a sense of well-being. This technique has also been employed successfully in maintaining states of hypnoanalgesia and anaesthesia for longer obstetrical and operative procedures, i.e., a Caesarian section was done utilizing no anaesthetics or analgesics. The patient responded beautifully. She felt no pain whatsoever and had an excellent postoperative recovery. She remained in the trance for over two hours until she received instructions for awakening. Since the above modification in this technique, I have had a high percentage of positive results in inducing and maintaining drugless sleep.

TECHNIQUE OF THE AUXILIARY HYPNOTIST

We have for some time been experimenting with the employment of an auxiliary third person, preferably a doctor, nurse, or a person with some prestige or authority in the eyes of the patient.

The positive responses of the patient to suggestion are strongly confirmed verbally by the auxiliary. For instance, the suggestion that "Your breathing has changed," is confirmed by the auxiliary with the remark, "There's already a marked change in the breathing."

The therapist may remark to the auxiliary, "The patient is relaxing very rapidly," and the auxiliary responds with the remark, "He's already showing signs of relaxation. It's remarkable."

This method has been most helpful in speeding up the induction and particularly when some degree of resistance is encountered. This method is especially adapted for use in teaching clinics where a larger group may be present. Further, it is of great value in a busy clinic with a large case load, because the time required for induction can often be markedly reduced by this procedure.

I have found that suggestions made via the medium of directing the remarks to a third person instead of the patient sometimes have an even greater suggestive effect since the patient feels that he is eavesdropping on a confidential, professional exchange of information about himself, a sort of privileged communication. This effect can be markedly reinforced by the conversation of the therapist and the auxiliary being affected in a whisper sufficiently audible for the patient to "overhear," as though it were not intended for him to hear.

SUMMARY DISCUSSION

I should like to clearly emphasize that the endogenic respiratory method is not, and should not, be based on hyperventilation.

The author has had one case thus far in which a patient being treated for nicotinism consciously, compulsively force-breathed while unconsciously resisting hypnotic induction. This patient began to show early signs of alkalotic tetany with the characteristic finger position and a feeling of numbness in his extremities. This was immediately terminated by strongly commanding the patient to hold his breath—thus causing an acid base shift and reducing blood alkalinity. The procedure bases solely on hypnotic suggestion. The subject is instructed to breathe slowly and deeply. No forced respiration is employed. Suggestions are given that the breathing is relaxing progressively as is the patient. Further, the slow deep respiration is not permitted to continue for more than several minutes. When longer periods are required for induction, one is obviously dealing with resistance. Such resistance should, of course, be promptly discussed and resolved wherever possible. If there is resistance to eye closure, it is often better to have the patient fixate on a point on the ceiling and apply the classical Braid-Liebeault method. I modify this by suggesting that Bell-brain reflex phenomena will then occur speeding up feelings of relaxation and drowsiness. If resistance continues, it is best to point out that the subject has not yet passed the test. Exploration of the patient's resistance should be promptly pursued.

Although Leitner and Weitzenhoffer have pointed to the observation that deep inspiration heightens suggestibility in patients, it has been my experience that the significant factor appears not to be the former, but rather the factor of maintaining marked concentration on the breathing rhythm. Often patients have been rapidly relaxed without even breathing deeply. Of course, the individual suggestibility of patients varies greatly.

The subject is instructed to the effect that he will be shown how to relax himself easily under the hypnotist's direction and supervision. As a result, the subject is put in the position of taking some initiative to obtain relaxation with the doctor's help. Thus, as previously noted, no attempt is made to dominate the patient but rather to assist him by showing him how he can voluntarily attain hypnotic relaxation.

This is a systemic procedure and differs radically from Schultz's autogenic training in which body parts are relaxed progressively in stages. The author feels that since hypnosis is based on a psychic suggestion mechanism, relaxation can be best and most rapidly effected through a central systemic method.

I have for some time felt that progressive relaxation methods of hypnotic induction are not only too time-consuming but generally impractical in a busy clinic setting. Further, prolonged procedures may increase resistance. This, of course, has not only resulted in a higher incidence of failures in initial hypnotic induction attempts but has in many instances markedly affected hypnotic transference and communication adversely. Hence, since it is conceded that hypnotic suggestion is a central psychic influence, I felt that it should be possible to rapidly induce patients by a centrally emanating total systemic procedure rather than piecemeal. Our clinical experience covering a large number of cases who were hypnotized by my method has completely supported the above conclusion. The percentage of successful primary induction was no less than 95 per cent.

In regard to the earlier efforts of Sargent and Fraser to induce hypnosis by means of hyperventilation, I should like to make the following comments: First, they were largely experimental and as such made a significant contribution. It is my opinion that forced breathing for purposes of induction is unnecessary and contraindicated. Not only is there a danger of gaseous alkalosis, but the resulting clouding of the psyche impairs communicability. Sargent and Fraser may have actually sought to induce a milder state of gaseous alkalosis and did not intend to hypnotize patients by suggestion. Nevertheless, their investigations represent a contribution of value. At any rate, they reported no use of suggestion in their induction procedure.

Many patients are willing to accept only a slight state of hypnotic relaxation during the first induction. They are feeling their way and are unwilling to surrender their conscious selves entirely.

It is best to let such a patient relax progressively. After several inductions, such patients can be hypnotized with great rapidity and often to a considerable depth.

It should be pointed out that under hypnosis, the hypersensitivity of the patient is marked. Thus, consideration of the patient's feelings and wishes should be carefully taken into account. The patient can be subject to considerable anxiety and emotional disturbance. Should this mount sufficiently in intensity, the patient will awaken as though from a frightening dream (nightmare).

As indicated earlier, it is advisable to run the aforementioned susceptibility tests prior to proceeding with hypnotic induction. When possible, it is best—after the initial susceptibility tests—to proceed with the endogenic three-step test and then take the subject deeper into the trance. It is most important to attach considerable significance to testing the patient prior to hypnotic induction. Furthermore, it is highly important to present the induction itself as a test, so that in the event of failure, it is the patient and not the doctor that has failed the test.

If a patient fails a susceptibility test, this does not necessarily mean he cannot be hypnotized. With many patients, the onset of heightened suggestibility is a step-by-step progressive one. For example, with reference to the hand clasp test mentioned earlier, if there are indications that a patient may not respond to an authoritarian style presentation of this test, because of an underlying resentment of authority or fear of loss of control, then a permissive style of the hand-clasp test procedure should be used: Ask the patient to raise his arms in a comfortable position, bent at the elbows, and to hold them over his lap with the fingers intertwined and the hands loosely clasped. Tell the patient, "As you sit there, look down at your hands as they are loosely clasped before you. Imagine that your hands are the paws of a vise, closing together tighter and tighter, (repeat), until soon you will undoubtedly notice signs of a gradual, although perhaps at first almost imperceptible inner tension developing as your fingers close down steadily tighter against your hands—until eventually they feel locked like a vise and you cannot open them—not even when I tell you to try to do so."

It has become clear on the basis of considerable clinical evidence that hypnotic suggestibility can be heightened when actual physical changes occur within the subject's body. It occurred to me that if the hypnotist could effect a change in the subject's physiology by means of hypnotic suggestion which could be observed by the subject, it would not only heighten suggestibility but could trigger off a kind of suggestive chain reaction which could greatly facilitate a progressively deepening hypnotic trance. This is accomplished in endogenic induction technique. Deep breathing produces the Hering-Breuer phenomena with the resulting reduction in breathing and apnoea changes which the subject can readily observe.

Chapter 5

MANIFESTATIONS AND HANDLING OF RESISTANCE TO HYPNOTIC INDUCTION

Although most normal persons, under favorable conditions, possess the capacity to be hypnotized, there are wide individual variances in susceptibility and resistance to hypnosis. If the resistance is conscious, it can usually be dealt with readily and resolved. More difficult is the handling of resistances on an unconscious level. Generally, these require working through and analysis for resolution. Some of the more common resistances have been discussed, such as fear of surrendering one's will, fear of dependency and loss of independent capacity for initiative and action, fear of loss of control and helplessness and of being overpowered, of being banned, fear of failure, defiance of authority and the need to prove one's self stronger. Defiance of authority relates to earlier defiance toward parents and teachers. Competitiveness is not certainly common in a competition society such as ours. Some such subjects see hypnotic induction as a contest of wills. Presenting hypnotic induction as a test for them to achieve helps to counter this power struggle.

One of the most common sources of resistance is the anxiety and embarrassment concerning the possible disclosure of conflicts which the individual is not yet willing to communicate. The resolution of resistance depends in a great measure upon the patient's capacity for insight and his ability to recognize the sources of his resistance and to discuss them in particular with the therapist. Most resistances can be overcome by providing a fuller insight and ventilation of the feelings and conflicts involved. Patience, gentle encouragement, and reassurance may often be very helpful. The ability of the therapist to calm and reassure a patient can be a decisive factor in overcoming resistance. Resourcefulness on the part of the hypnotist can be employed as, for example, Weitzenhoffer's procedure for dealing with feelings of defiance and the need of the subject to prove himself superior to the hypnotist.

In such instances, the subject is prepared by being told that considerable intelligence and concentrative ability are necessary for anyone to be hypnotized, which is the opposite of what prospective subjects are usually told. The various suggestions are then given in a way which challenges the subject's ability to perform satisfactorily. For example, note Wolberg's procedure, which states: "You do not command him to make his arm stiff and rigid, or even tell him that his arm is becoming so." Instead, say something like, "See if you can make your arm stiff and rigid so that you cannot bend it. It takes such effort and concentration to do this. Let's see if you have the necessary ability to do so." This desire on the part of the subject to prove himself can be further utilized to therapeutic advantage and as an ego-strengthening device.

I have often found that, while inducing a patient in front of a colleague, a remark such as: "This patient is intelligent enough to understand the instructions and carry them out;" or, "This is one of my best patients and she is intelligent enough to cooperate—you see that she is already responding beautifully" is effective. At this point, the colleague previously has been instructed to remark: "It is quite remarkable. This patient is relaxing beautifully." At times it is necessary to utilize signs of resistance in a suggestive manner such as: "Your eyelids are now flicking. This is typical of what happens just before deeper relaxation. You are doing fine." Reassurances of this type can be repeated several times. I heartily agree with Erickson that attempts to overpower or influence the patient against his own desire or will may often result in greater resistance and is generally contraindicated. The projections of the patient can be manipulated in such a manner as to serve the hypnotherapeutic objective. Erickson suggests that acceptance and utilization of the subject's responses, regardless of their nature, to further trance behavior makes for more effective hypnosis. The fact that a subject volunteers to be hypnotized and simultaneously offers resistance is evidence of an ambivalence which, once recognized, can be made to serve the purposes of both the hypnotist and the subject.

Ambivalence towards induction is best dealt with by conveying to the subject the impression that ambivalent feelings are part of the usual experience associated with induction. In this manner the ambivalence may be utilized to further trance induction. Erickson and Wolberg have skillfully utilized this approach.

The patient is in effect made to feel that his resistance has been unmasked by the sharp insight of the hypnotist and strong suggestion is used that he will go into hypnotic sleep in spite of the fact that he is resisting it. His eyes or attention can be fixated and the suggestion employed that the more he resists, the more difficult it will be for the subject to keep from falling asleep. The following is an example of Wolberg's technique in dealing with ambivalence.

"As you sit here looking into my eyes, you begin to resist falling asleep. You say to yourself, "It isn't possible to fall asleep. I can't fall asleep. But you will find that the more you resist, the more difficult it is to keep from falling asleep. The harder you fight, the sleepier you get. Try it, and you will see that the more you resist falling asleep, the sleepier you are. Fight hard against falling asleep. Try not to fall asleep, and the harder you try, the sleepier you get. The more you fight, the sleepier you get. Fight hard to keep awake. Try to defy me, try to keep awake; but the more you defy me, the sleepier you get. Your eyelids are getting heavier and heavier until they close." By such means, the ambivalence can be employed to deepen the trance.

I have often found that helping the patient to gain insight into the causes of their ambivalence and the senselessness of such often resolves the resistance. A good example is that of a 52-year old woman who was suffering from chronic bronchitis and early emphysema. She was a career person, very independent, rigid and highly fearful of giving up control. She conceded the latter trait quite frankly. She admitted that she enjoyed smoking but realized that her bronchitis and emphysema were worsening. It was then discovered that she had a marked anxiety of asphyxiation and of becoming a helpless invalid. After a frank discussion in which she recognized the importance of cooperation, she submitted to hypnosis and hypnoaversion treatment of her tobacco compulsion was successfully achieved.

Erickson emphasizes that the behavioral responses of the patient himself serve as a basis for suggestion. He points out that resistance is best utilized by creating a situation in which it serves a specific purpose. This may be accomplished by wording the suggestions in such a manner that no matter what the subject does or does not do, he is made to feel that he actually is responding according to plan and as the hypnotist desires. I have found Erickson's suggestion of great value.

Weitzenhoffer, in discussing the hand levitation method demonstrates his method of utilizing the various responses of the subject as follows: "In essence, we told the subject that one of his hands would do something. Maybe it would press down, or possibly it would move upward, or still again it might do nothing at all. The subject was told that he might feel a tingling in his hand, or maybe a sensation of warmth, but surely something would happen. Possibly, he was told, it would be a twitching of the muscles of his hands, or perhaps a finger. Perhaps the middle finger would move, or maybe the little finger—possibly the whole hand. And so forth."

Weitzenhoffer points out that in this manner all possible reactions to the suggestions are included under the label of a satisfactory response without any specific commitments on the part of the hypnotist. Thus, even resistance manifestations can be treated as constructive cooperative responses. Erickson also suggests that all resistance should be localized as much as possible upon irrelevant alternatives. For example, one can suggest to a subject resisting hand levitation that his right hand will move upward, but that the left one will not. Erickson further emphasizes that one should never attempt to correct the subject's behavior, change it, or compel him to produce a response. This may often stimulate resistance.

Watkins expresses the view that in order to successfully handle resistance and the ambivalent feelings of the patient, it is necessary to have a fuller and more intimate understanding of the personality structure, the transference needs, ego defenses and the cathexes, the emotional attachments of the patient. In addition, he points out: "It would further require that the hypnotist be quite aware of his own countertransference needs, role abilities and limitations." Watkins, in discussing the significance of transference in hypnosis, points out transference reactions of different orders may be associated with different levels of hypnosis on the same subject. That the inability of the subject to develop a trance depth beyond a certain point may simply reflect a change in his transference needs as induction has progressed. Thus, the new need of the patient can be satisfied and hence greater depth obtained only if the hypnotist takes on a different transference role. For instance, a relative degree of passivity and permissiveness on the part of the hypnotist may yield best results at one stage of induction whereas, at another, a strong authoritative approach may be indicated.

In some instances, a specific type of transference may be ineffectual at any level since it does not meet with the basic transference needs of the patient. To illustrate, I should like to cite a case of a middle-aged woman who was seeking treatment for nicotinism. Upon initial interview, she revealed mixed feelings about terminating smoking. Hypnotic induction was first attempted by the author's endogenic method which permits the subject to retain some degree of initiative. Despite some effort on her part, she was unable to attain the trance state. She described her feelings as being "on the verge but not completely relaxed." At this point, the author suddenly altered his approach and gave a strong command without warning— "sleep." This was combined with a pass of the hand over the subject's eyes. The patient promptly went into a trance. This case illustrates the importance of assessing the transference needs of the patient and rapidly altering the induction approach.

Meares describes a method for dealing with negativistic subjects, inducing hypnosis by repetitive movements of the arm. He holds the arm by the cuff or wrist and moves it back and forth, simultaneously suggesting: "Your arm goes back and forth, back and forth, your arm goes back and forth, back and forth. Your arm automatically goes back and forth, automatically back and forth. . . ." After a short while, the negativistic subject will tend to spontaneously move his arm opposite to the direction suggested each time. When this happens, according to Meares, the patient is hypnotized.

In cases in which the difficulty in concentration is the form of resistance encountered, Wolberg recommends using the counting technique. Once the patient is comfortably seated and asked to fixate upon an object or to look straight ahead of him at the wall, he is told: "I am going to count and I want you to follow me closely. When I say 'one,' you will close your eyes and keep them closed until I say 'two.' When I say 'two' you will open your eyes. Then when I say 'three,' you will close them again and keep them closed until I say 'four.' Do you understand? (If the subject seems to show some confusion, you can demonstrate for him what you want. Some hypnotists make it a standard practice to demonstrate these instructions while giving them.) You will keep on opening and closing your eyes as I count until they get very tired. You will find yourself becoming more and more drowsy and sleepy. After awhile your eyes will have become so-o-o heavy and you will be so-o-o sleepy that your eyes will close and remain closed and you will go into a deep, sound sleep. You will have no desire to open your eyes, you will want to sleep, to sleep deeply and soundly."

The hypnotist then begins to count in a monotonous voice, pausing after each number at the rate of one or two numbers per second, meanwhile watching the subject's reactions closely. By observing the subject's reaction to the count, for instance; if he consistently anticipates the count especially on opening his eyes, he is very likely not paying close attention or resisting. On the other hand, if he has difficulty opening his eyes or keeping them open, he is likely to be entering into a hypnotic trance. In this manner it is possible to have some indicator of the progress of the trance induction. The hypnotic effect can be further intensified by using suggestions of drowsiness, heaviness of the eyelids, and sleep between the counts. Weitzenhoffer points out that the subject in some cases may continue to open and close his eyes despite becoming deeply hypnotized and that this is due to the fact that the subject does not clearly understand the instructions, or that each count acts through association as a command suggestion. He further describes termination of induction as follows: when it appears that the subject is hypnotized, "Wait until he closes his eyes again, then stop counting and say something like 'now your eyes are closed and you are deep asleep. Your eyes are very heavy . . . like lead. They are stuck fast . . . so fast that you cannot open them.' " Specifically, the subject is told not to open his eyes until the next count but he is not told to close them before the next count. Weitzenhoffer points out this is because he may fall into a deep trance and his eyes may close anytime in the induction. It is obvious that adding conditions for eye closure at this point may interfere with induction. The above procedure illustrates the great importance of specific and careful wording when giving suggestions.

There are, of course, numerous methods for attempting to intensify concentration such as that of the classical metronome procedure and other methods which employ a rhythmic sound or movement. The author agrees with Brown that the rate of rhythm which works best is that which is adjusted to bodily rhythm such as pulse beat or respiration. Other standard procedures based on the same general principle are those of the pendulum and rotating mirror method, hypnodisks and similar devices.

INITIAL SIGNS OF RESISTANCE

Some early signs of possible resistance to hypnotic induction are:

a. Forgetting appointment, skipping of appointments or coming late. Some new patients get lost in spite of clearcut instructions on how to get to office.

b. Restlessness and general uneasiness, procrastination.

c. Trembling—smoking—going to the bathroom, etc.

d. Repeated questioning and scepticism prior to induction, irritability.

e. Complaints of trouble relaxing. Such patients often suffer from insomnia.

f. Silence or excessive verbosity, i.e., talking during early phase of induction.

g. The patient may say, "I don't really want to quit smoking, drinking, etc. My being here is my wife's or my husband's idea."

h. Resistance to eye closure.

i. Lack of compliance, virtually ignoring instructions during induction.

j. Resistance to taking deep breaths, i.e., negativism may be indicated if patient is told to breathe deeply and does not comply or does the opposite.

k. Blocking on accepting suggestions, i.e., that the breathing is getting shallower or the hand is getting lighter. (If patient continues this too long, instruct patient to stop breathing and hold his breath. If he still does not comply, cover the nose and mouth with gauze or tissue for a moment, telling him that it is necessary to reduce his oxygen intake to prevent any alkalotic tetanie reactions.)

The patient may try to test himself by trying to maintain control over bodily movements. He may voluntarily try to move fingers, to flick his eyelids or open them, to try to move his lips or swallow, or to move his arm or head to test his controls. (Note: At this point, it is important to suggest that such movements will take him deeper.)

RESISTANCE AND ANXIETY

Resistance to induction is usually associated with anxiety. If the patient doesn't relax with calming and reassuring suggestion plus lifting and dropping of his arms, it is best to tell him that before he can pass the induction test, it would be better for him to discuss what is troubling him.

RESISTANCE AND EYE CLOSURE

In the event of opening his eyes, he should be told that he will keep his eyelids closed so that his eyes won't dry out and burn. Furthermore, he should be warned that the longer he keeps his eyes closed, the more comfortable, drowsy and relaxed he will feel.

Interestingly, patients who carry out this post hypnotic instruction usually respond favorably to the treatment.

While premature, spontaneous opening of the eyelids may be due to resistance, in some instances it is due to the hypnotist failing to emphasize that "Your eyes will remain closed until I give you instructions to reopen them" or that the patient misunderstands an instruction and believes that the session is terminated.

If the resistance is persistent, then it is best to suggest that the patient will awaken fully at the count of 30 (counting from 20 to 30) and that the next time he is instructed to relax, he will be able to relax much deeper. It is always best to resolve the cause of the resistance as soon as possible.

RESISTANCE AND FEAR OF LOSING CONTROL

The most common cause of resistance to hypnotic induction is the fear of loss of conscious control and a dread of helplessness. For example, a man in his early 40's revealed such resistance, which he recognized after some discussion as a subconscious fear of loss of control. It was suggested that the fear could perhaps be resolved after a few sessions. He soon revealed that during his preadolescence he had a rather severe bedwetting problem. On one occasion, at nine years of age, he was ridiculed and humiliated by his mother in front of his friends. He began to increasingly dread the loss of control over his bladder. This fear was repressed. He had been aware that he had a fear of helplessness which he felt when up in an airplane or out on a small boat in deep water. His dread of hypnosis became clear to him in terms of being helpless and overpowered. After some discussion, his fear of hypnosis disappeared.

With patients who are rather fearful of losing control, it is often best to use the following approach.

"I'm going to show you how you can relax yourself. You won't relinquish control unless you really want to. You have arranged this treatment session. It is all your own initiative and all I can do is help you to accomplish what you desire. So let me give you the instructions, which you then give yourself." The patient is taking the first phase of deep breathing and relaxation and then the count begins. "Now you will count silently to yourself as I count, putting yourself under. After you have put yourself under and are going deeper and deeper, I shall show you how you can go much deeper with very little effort." Actually, if desired, the patient can silently repeat all the instructions from the beginning—going progressively deeper and deeper.

TRANCE DEEPENING AND DEALING WITH RESISTANCE

Not infrequently upon the initial induction, the patient will go into a light trance but will not comply with suggestions that his hand is elevating (hand levitation). At this point, the hypnotist should suggest that, "It seems that you have relaxed so deeply that you are unable to raise your hand, so I'm going to help you and put it on your forehead, so that you can receive a very pleasant hypnotic transfusion which will take you deeper. You will soon feel limp and very deeply relaxed and your left hand will begin to fall as you will no longer be able to hold it up. Your left hand is falling . . . (repeat suggestion.)" If the hand does not fall and the patient resists the suggestion, it suggests strong resistance to induction and resistance to loss of conscious control.

You can tell the patient, "I'm going to test your arm to see if you are so deep that you can't bring your hand down," suggesting that as "you drop your arm, you will fall off deeper." If the patient continues to resist the arm drop and maintains tension in the arm muscles, then tell the patient, "You haven't yet passed the test and it would be best to discuss the reasons for your not allowing yourself to pass the test." However, if the arm falls limply, that is a good indication. The trance can then be deepened by progressive relaxation, dropping one extremity after another, repeatedly suggesting greater hypnotic relaxation and limpness. This can also be done by dropping the same arm repeatedly until it is completely limp.

I have found that when hand levitation is not occurring in response to suggestion, there are two procedures that can be attempted:

1. Have the subject press down with his right hand giving the suggestion that as the right presses down, the left hand elevates. If resistance is marked and hand levitation does not occur on repeated suggestion, then it is best to proceed to step 2.

2. The suggestion is given that the patient has gone under so deeply that he cannot raise his arm and therefore "I (the hypnotist) will lift your hand for you and place it on your forehead so that you can get a deep hypnotic transfusion which will take you deeper and deeper." Usually, the subject's hand then drops as the suggestion is given, "You will become deeply relaxed and your left hand will become limp and heavy and fall like a dead weight, causing you to fall off deeper."

The subject can be then taken even deeper by suggesting that pressure would be applied to the hypnotic centers in the brain (hypnotist compressing both temples) and "You will become even much more deeply relaxed."

In many subjects a paradoxical response can be evoked by suggesting, "The more you try to open your eyes, the tighter they'll close or the more you push down with your right hand, the more the left hand will rise."

Another auxiliary deepening procedure that can be used at this point is to take hold of the wrist and rotate the whole arm in a circle slowly suggesting that "each turn will take you deeper." As the patient relaxes, the arm gets hypotonic and when the arm is heavy and limp, it is dropped with the suggestion that as it falls you will fall off deeper.

In some instances, where there is resistance to hand levitation, the hypnotist can place his fingertips on the fingertips of the patient's hand, suggesting, "I am going to measure the rate of lifting of your hand." Then the hypnotist withdraws his fingers slowly and gives the suggestion that the fingers of the patient have moved away from the hand.

If the patient spontaneously emerges from the trance opening his eyes, it is best to discuss why he opened his eyes. What was on his mind? Was anything troubling him? Was he afraid? Patients reveal such reasons as fears of loss of control, fears of being abused, of revealing something they feel guilty or ashamed about or just simply being curious about a new experience. Others confess they had heard bad things about hypnosis, etc., about people under being made to do something they didn't wish to. There are, of course, instances when the subject simulates being hypnotized and sooner or later opens his eyes. In any case, a frank discussion of his reactions is indicated.

RESISTANCE AS DEFIANCE

A very common cause of resistance is subconscious defiance. Numerous patients have been able to recognize that their resistance paralleled the defiance they had felt toward an overly strict and demanding parent or teacher in adolescence. Such resistance is often manifest in individuals undergoing treatment for drinking, smoking or overeating. These persons often relive the earlier disapproval of their parents and their resentful defiance at being denied and criticized. They are unaware that they are at cross purposes regarding the treatment and insight into their behavior may be very helpful.

DISCUSSING RESISTANCE WITH THE PATIENT

When there is manifest resistance, it is best to advise one or two sessions or more to discuss the patient's resistance. It is best to avoid the word "resistance" as this may have a different meaning for the patient than for the therapist. The patient will often protest by saying in a hurt fashion,

"I wasn't resisting. I was really trying. I wouldn't have come to you if I didn't want the treatment." The hypnotist makes a comment, "You haven't been able to pass the test yet and comply with the instructions. I know you must really desire to, so I'm going to give you another chance if you really want to."

It is better to discuss why the patient had difficulties and couldn't pass the test, so that the next time they will have no difficulty. Such sessions will usually help to resolve resistance by the developing of good rapport, the necessary insights, and thereby reducing anxiety. That is, once the anxieties or disturbed feelings are ventilated, the patient usually has no further difficulty in relaxing.

POSTHYPNOTIC SUGGESTION

The depth of the hypnotic state, the degree of suggestibility and compliance can be readily determined by giving posthypnotic suggestions, for example, "After awakening, you will count quickly from one to ten, but you will omit the number nine. You will be sure to omit the number nine." Patients in a light trance because of a resistance conflict may not omit the number nine. Frequently, to determine the effectiveness of the aversion treatment given to a cigarette smoker, the patient will be given the instruction following the treatment that, if he has any cigarettes on his person, he will leave them on your desk and will forget that he left them there. Compliance is also a good prognostic indicator.

RESISTANCE IN ENDOGENIC METHOD OF INDUCTION

As stated before, in the endogenic method resistance can be very readily detected. The patient simply does not comply with the instructions to breathe deeply. He either hesitates on following instructions or breathes in a shallow manner, and often he does both. With the Braid optic fixation method, the subject usually will avoid fixation of his eyes and will either deviate his eyes or open and close them.

The endogenic procedure has the advantage of providing an excellent indicator of the degree of cooperation, resistance and relaxation of the patient.

The patient who is cooperative will immediately hyperventilate and concentrate on his breathing as instructed. The resistive patient will usually fail to do this. On occasion, when queried, they may offer some reason for not breathing such as, "I can't breathe deeply, Doctor—it hurts!" or "It makes me cough," or "I'm afraid." If the patient has a respiratory condition, it is best to have him breathe lightly and put emphasis on progressive muscle relaxation and hand levitation as a prime induction factor.

Since the patient has been told that as he relaxes, his breathing will become easier, shallower, and relaxed, the changes in respiration provide an excellent indicator of degree of relaxation.

When continued deep breathing occurs, the patient is clearly having difficulty in relaxing and is compulsively trying to force himself to relax. This should be terminated and an effort to explore the problem made.

Another indication of unconscious resistance is the patient's admission that he is having difficulty in concentrating on his breathing.

In any case, the basis of the resistance should always immediately be probed before any attempt is made to procede further. Anxieties can usually be resolved after the cause is determined. Sometimes minor resistance can be overcome but such patients in the initial phases of treatment usually do not reach the same depth of hypnosis as non-resistive patients.

Summary Discussion

Resistance in hypnosis is most frequently based on:

1. Fear of surrender of will and authority to an external authority
2. Fear of the new unknown (magical) experience (popular superstitions about hypnosis)
3. Fear of appearing ridiculous because of association with magic, sideshow
4. Fear of the real motives of the hypnotist
5. Fear of not being able to reawaken, fear of death
6. Fear of dependence
7. Fear of loss of control and helplessness often encountered in insomniacs associated with fears of injury and death
8. Fear of revealing strongly repressed conflicts and affectivity
9. Situational resistance, "I have an appointment and I'm afraid I'll be late," or "I can't stand anyone (people) looking at me when I'm trying to relax or go to sleep." (Note: It is often necessary to let such patients relax while alone.) "I need to go to the toilet, etc."
10. Fear of one's own affectivity—fear of loss of ego-control. Fear of being exposed—revealed).
11. Resistance against recalling painful past experiences
12. Hostile feelings towards the hypnotist and resistance to his voice and manner
13. Shame or guilt feelings
14. Resistance to the respiratory method of induction in certain patients suffering from respiratory anxiety may occur.

Not infrequently, these may be related to an organic cardiac or pulmonary condition. Such patients often become quite concerned about their breathing and frequently tend to restrict their respiration. Any conscious effort at obeying the therapist's instructions to breathe deeply may be met with anxiety of varying intensity and both conscious and unconscious resistance. Many individuals tend to correlate heavy deep respiration with heart failure, pneumonia, particularly if they have witnessed terminal breathing of a dying person. Frequently, earlier repressed childhood anxieties are activated.

In such cases, it would be wise to explore and resolve the anxiety. If possible, resistances should be dealt with consciously through discussion. The hypnotist should not be too energetic but permit the patient to warm up to him and establish rapport.

Resistance is also manifest by:

1. Resisting and noncooperative during induction attempt
2. Rationalizations of evasive type
3. Relinquishing only part of ego-maintaining the watchdog ego, because of anxiety and distrust, therefore resisting deeper hypnotic trance, becoming the observer rather than the participant
4. Resistance often manifest by struggling to come out of trance rather than trying to stay in. In some instances, there can be resistance to consciousness as well as to hypnosis.
5. Interesting type of resistance is patient's insistance that he hadn't been hypnotized after being brought out of the trance. He wants to remind the hypnotist that he hadn't really surrendered.
6. Posthypnotic resistance to carrying out instructions following emergence from trance, i.e., such as arranging the next appointment

RELATIONSHIP OF COMPULSIVITY AND FEAR TO RESISTANCE

In general, compulsive types of patients may manifest greater resistance to hypnosis. Patients who tend to present obsessive-compulsive symptoms similarly may have difficulty in falling asleep. These patients, on analysis of their difficulties, present deep-seated fears of being injured, attacked, of dying, etc. Such patients may remark that they are afraid to give up consciousness because they fear loss of conscious control. Some fear not being able to reawaken. Here sleep or hypnosis may be unconsciously equated with dying or becoming helpless and vulnerable to injury and attack. Such patients often fear and resent the state of relative passive helplessness experienced in sleep or hypnosis. In my opinion, compulsive behavior usually represents an unconscious defense against repressed fears.

Recently, we had such a compulsive patient. A young man came in stating that he wanted to give up smoking. An attempt was made to relax him by the endogenic method. However, he did not follow the specific instructions to breathe slowly and deeply but immediately began to force-breathe rapidly. This he continued to do in spite of the instructions to stop force-breathing. As his breathing began to take on a character similar to Cheyne-Stokes and his fingers formed into the position characteristic of a Tetanie cramp, it was decided to very energetically intervene, and loudly command him to hold his breath repeatedly. He was finally persuaded to hold his breath. I was ready to use gauze to cut off his oxygen supply for a short time in order to relieve the patient's state of gaseous alkalosis. The patient recovered rapidly, was bewildered, and a bit confused for several minutes. Later, he explained that he didn't really desire to stop smoking, that he enjoyed it too much, and that he was trying to force himself to comply. He added that he often would discipline himself in a compulsive manner in order to make himself do what he didn't really wish to do. I advised him that it wasn't wise to force himself to submit to treatment for this would only create inner conflict and a poor therapeutic result.

In my opinion, prolonged hyperventilation is definitely contraindicated and unnecessary for purposes of induction. This procedure is not only hazardous, but of little therapeutic value, since the patient thus induced has a clouded sensorium and his communicability is markedly reduced. Deep breathing should be stopped by commanding the patient to relax his breathing, hold his breath, or stop deep breathing. If he doesn't comply, as said before, it is best to put gauze over his mouth and nose briefly in order to prevent development of alkalosis and tetanie. The patient should be told that the moist gauze is being put on his mouth and nose to help him feel better. Generally, on induction, I instruct the patients to breathe deeply but slowly.

I have found further that patients who have authoritarian personalities and possess a strong need to dominate are the very ones who will resist submission to hypnosis most. Such patients often have inner fears of being attacked, overpowered, or being helpless. Furthermore, I have observed that markedly masculine aggressive women may often resist being hypnotized. Frequently, they try to compete with the therapist and prove that he can't overpower them. This is often an unconscious game of contest of wills of which the patient may be totally unaware. It is a game that the therapist must never enter into. Rather, he must clarify his position to the patient. "To accomplish what you desire we must work together. I can and will only do what you desire me to. I will only carry out your wish. You, therefore, have nothing to fight against or worry about." Good results are only achieved by cooperation.

Resistance can also be differentiated into that directed against external influence and that directed against autosuggestion.

The number of persons resistant to autosuggestive or modified combined techniques is minimal.

In general, when resistance is encountered, the first step is not to press the issue. This may intensify anxiety and resistance, sometimes to a panic level.

The next point is to begin the analysis of resistance. There are a number of ways to lessen anxiety, heighten suggestibility and resistance:

1. By telling the patient that the purpose of the session is to test his capacity to relax or test a physiological function (respiration, eye muscle, muscle relaxation, strength, etc.)

2. Suggestions can be given prior to or during the test procedure. Examples: For patients who are resisting influence of others, encourage self-relaxation exercise. Emphasize clearly that the hypnotist will only help him to achieve his objective.

3. It is sometimes possible to relax patients in stages when resistance is encountered, although this procedure is time-consuming and at times unsuccessful. It is generally better to attempt no induction until proper rapport is established and resistance is resolved.

4. Use of auxiliary hypnotist to combat resistance and intensify suggestion.

5. Sometimes it is important to evaluate suggestibility of patient. This can be done by having the patient put his feet together with his eyes closed and standing at attention, and suggest that he is beginning to sway. Another method to have patient extend arms parallel and with eyes closed and suggest that one arm is falling.

6. Avoid use of term "hypnosis" in the beginning. Substitute the term "pleasant relaxation."

It is beneficial to create the anticipation of pleasurable relaxation. It is important to discuss the question of the resistance patients show to awakening from trance. This is usually an indication of conscious tensions and psychic suffering, that reality is disturbing and painful to the patient. The reasons for these feelings should be probed into. In such instances, the patient may actually desire escape from the reality situation.

Most susceptible are patients with a high degree of autosuggestibility. It follows that they can also be more readily influenced by suggestive therapy.

FEAR OF HELPLESSNESS

As mentioned, a common form of resistance encountered is the belief of the patient that hypnosis will render him helpless. Certain patients have intense dread of helplessness. Such patients usually experience anxiety prior to sleep since they are often disturbed by threatening fantasies of being hurt, overpowered, or helpless. They often reexperience difficulty in relaxing and falling asleep. It is unwise to attempt hypnotic induction in such instances until these anxieties are allayed. When there is unresolved anxiety the closer the patient gets to losing control, the more panicked and resistive he becomes.

OTHER FACTORS INFLUENCING HYPNOTIC SUGGESTIBILITY

Environmental stimuli: Suggestion may be enhanced by providing a monotonous low-grade sound, diminished light, constantly moving object, metronome, pendulum, revolving disc, etc.

Religion: The religious beliefs of some patients that it is sinful to permit another power outside of God to control one may be circumvented by telling the patient that he receives instructions which he will follow so that he can relax himself into hypnosis. Yet, religious persons are usually very prone to suggestive influence and generally make excellent subjects. That is to say, usually devout believers, fervent patriots, and conformists are good subjects.

Sex: I have found no significant difference when working with larger numbers of patients as regards the susceptibility to hypnosis of male as compared to female patients. For some, the sex of the hypnotist may certainly be a factor. With the endogenic method which involves physiological changes as well as suggestion, it appears to me that a lesser degree of rapport needs to be established *a priori*. The matter of being able to surrender control appears to be the important consideration. The handling of loss of control fear is discussed in Chapter 11.

POSTHYPNOTIC SUGGESTION

Posthypnotic suggestion remains effective in my opinion only as long as the suggestion or command remains submerged in the unconscious and there is not too much inner resistance. Whether the influence remains depends also on the resistance that the patient feels against the posthypnotic suggestion. The influence is usually lost when it is recalled or brought to conscious awareness. Posthypnotic suggestions can be reinforced by repetition in subsequent hypnotic sessions. Suggestion can be used to help block conscious recall.

APPROACH TO INDUCTION

In resistive or anxious patients, this should seldom be direct. The patient, as said before, is presented with the possibility of practicing relaxation or testing his relaxation capacity—or another approach such as this is often effective, "Would you like me to show you how you can relax yourself when you feel nervous or uncomfortable or can't rest?" Always the source of the resistance should be explored as a first step.

Although some patients resist the idea of an external influence they may not feel similarly about inducing relaxation by themselves. More often, in such cases, I have the patient participate in the induction by counting with me, etc.

I have found it very effective to tell the patient that he is just being tested initially, then telling him that he has passed the test successfully and is now able to go deeper without difficulty. Thus, there is no interruption and the patient is taken progressively deeper into the trance.

In some instances, the subject will follow through with the instructions given by the hypnotist except that he will not, or cannot, concentrate on other instances. Patients sometimes create psychic diversions by trying to turn their attention away from the hypnotist to some other preoccupation.

HANDLING OF RESISTANCE

The author does not believe in trying to hypnotize patients who are not ready to accept hypnotic relaxation. I have in some instances hypnotized somewhat resistive juvenile delinquents and adult offenders at correctional institutions for purposes of investigating the background of an offense committed or to determine where a dangerous weapon had been concealed. Sometimes this requires outwitting ego defenses. In such instances the best method is an indirect one and may begin with simulating a medical examination and then an eye check. The hypnotist must here proceed with strong authoritativeness.

He instructs the patient that he is testing the eye muscles and the strength of fixation and convergence. This procedure is based on the Bell reflex. When the eyes are turned up, the upward lids cannot close. He is told to fixate his eyes on an object and to follow the object as it is placed far above his forehead. He is given strong suggestions to fixate on the object. As he is well fixated on the object, he is told that he will try to close his eyelids but that he cannot because he is in a hypnotic state; however he will recover the use of his eyelids after he has emerged from the trance. The hypnotist gently closes his eyes with the suggestion that, "You will now relax deeper and deeper. As you breathe deeply, now you will relax deeper and deeper and feel very comfortable."

In cases of very resistive patients, it is often best to use sodium amytal in conjunction with hypnotic suggestion. (Narcohypnosis).

THE ENDOGENIC METHOD

Generally, with the endogenic method, most subjects can be more readily hypnotized by a brief, logical, reasonable explanation of the physiological mechanisms of relaxation. We generally prefer to use the term relaxation rather than hypnosis. It has been our practice, in certain instances, where the endogenic method has failed, to attempt to relax the patient by having him gaze at an object on the ceiling (a method favored by Weitzenhoffer). The patient is told that he will soon experience the effects of the Bell Brain Reflex in which the eyeballs are rotated upwardly, the pupils become smaller and the eyelids descend and close, all accompanied by marked feelings of drowsiness. This latter method has succeeded in a fairly high percentage of people who would not respond to the endogenic method. This procedure generally requires more time and, in some instances, the hypnotist must be patient and permit the subject sufficient time for induction.

SOME CASE EXAMPLES OF RESISTANCE

As stated before, resistance is promptly manifest in the endogenic procedure by a failure to breathe deeply when so instructed. One patient complied, in part, giving up some degree of consciousness but remaining on guard, sort of subconsciously alert in a kind of hypnoidal type of relaxation which is characteristic of the sleep of certain animals, kind of defensive adaptation mechanism of the sleep function. When asked why he would not permit himself to relax completely, he said. "The doctors put something on that burnt arm of mine the other day and they said it wasn't going to hurt but it hurt awful bad and I was scared you were going to do something to me." When reassured, he relaxed promptly.

Another patient, who also manifested resistance not only by failing to follow the breathing instructions but also by not closing her eyes was a middle-aged woman. When asked whether she had any anxiety, she promptly remarked that she was afraid to give up the conscious state because she was afraid that she might not reawaken. This patient suffered from severe insomnia because of deep-seated fears of death. It later came out, under hypnosis, that she had a cancer phobia which had been created when she had asked a doctor why she had persistent stomach discomfort and a feeling of epigastric nausea. He replied that often the early manifestations of cancer appeared in this way. Her anxiety mounted and since then she had suffered from severe insomnia and anxiety.

At this point it is necessary to warn against failing to recognize the high degree of suggestibility which most patients have in the presence of a medical authority during the wakeful state. Unaware, doctors may make what appear to be offhand statements which have a seriously disturbing effect on the patient.

Since the doctor is dedicated to relieving rather than creating suffering, he must be aware of the tremendous power of suggestion that is his as an expert authority. He can, of course, similarly use offhand comments in a manner very beneficial to the patient.

I have found concerning the employment of suggestion, indirect suggestion methods by far the most effective both when a patient is under hypnosis or in the wakeful state. The patient is usually convinced that anything which he hears by means of eavesdropping on the doctor's conversation about him with his nurse, his colleagues, or members of his intimate family represents the real opinion of the doctor, and what the doctor really thinks is of paramount importance to most patients. When a patient eavesdrops, moreover, his ego defenses are down, for, after all, there is nothing to guard against. He is convinced that he is picking up "tidbits" of truth which he may feel are being withheld from him, and of course, that he must know what the doctor thinks. At any rate, he manages to often overhear these comments, frequently not even knowing that they concern him until they have been uttered. This is also why whispering in the ear of a patient in group hypnosis may have a strong suggestive effect. It must be important if it is withheld from others.

On the other hand, since patients are highly suggestive in such a situation, they are also very vulnerable and can be seriously harmed by a disturbing or frightening remark.

In order to further communication and provoke a response, I have had occasion to frequently utilize this technique in a provocative manner, both during the wakeful state and under hypnosis. I recall the case of a young woman whom I had selected for purposes of demonstration to the staff of the Wagner-Juaregg Clinic while in Vienna. She had made a serious suicide attempt and was quite depressed, agitated, and uncommunicative. I relaxed her into a trance without much difficulty; however, she still remained uncommunicative about her central problems and conflicts. At this point I conferred with her psychiatrist and instructed her to tell me what she could of the patient's background in a low voice but loud enough so that the patient in the trance could feel that she was eavesdropping. I further asked the doctor to make a few intentional distortions. This her psychiatrist did beautifully, and one could observe how intently the patient was following the verbal exchange. After the first distortion which was quite loaded and to the effect that she had apparently willfully rejected a certain young man's love and that she now regretted it, her face became quite flushed and she exclaimed—"No, that's a lie, doctor, it wasn't like that at all, please let me explain!"

The patient then had an extensive verbal and affective catharsis which proved to be of marked therapeutic benefit in the further treatment of her suicidal depression. The whole story of how her love had been spurned by a desirable young man and the resultant feelings of inadequacy and deep resentment at self poured out accompanied by strong affect and copious tears.

WHAT TO LOOK FOR IN THE REFRACTOR SUBJECT

It is essential to discover the cause of the refraction and remove it. Sometimes one thing, and then another, will cause the seemingly willing person to resist hypnosis.

Is the light suitable? The temperature comfortable? The chair or couch comfortable? Is a visit to the toilet necessary? Is there a disturbing noise? Odour? Does the patient have an appointment to keep? Or does the subject have suconscious fears which have not been removed or explained? After considering all of these aspects and any other possibilities then given, there should be a reevaluation of the methods, more specific instructions about hypnosis being an interpersonal relationship, in which the hypnotist and the subject produce the hypnotic state by cooperating. The refraction can be on a conscious or subconscious level. Latent fears of losing control, of doing or saying something unseemly or damaging may exist. Or he may be trying too hard, instead of just relaxing and "letting it happen." The tense, anxious person often makes this mistake, and it is the responsibility of the hypnotist to find a way to eliminate this difficulty. Sometimes the patient strives to be the observer rather than the subject. When queried, he may admit that he was curious and had been wondering about the secret of hypnosis for a long time.

REEVALUATION OF METHODS

One approach to overcoming refraction is to start over again with the waking suggestions. Observe carefully the reaction to the two different approaches—the permissive and the authoritarian. Execute several permissive and then, several authoritarian techniques, and note the difference, if any, in the response. A classic example of improper application of technique is the following: the subject seems rather dazed, eyes wide, rather fearful, even a glazed look in the eyes, and expresses great eagerness to be hypnotized. This subject is already partially under hypnosis just through the expectation of being hypnotized. The operator applies a long drawn-out technique, like progressive relaxation, followed by a long count, a slow, (permissive, lullaby-type of talk) and finds that nothing is happening . . .

nothing favorable, that is. The subject loses his tension, relaxes a little, and suddenly loses his suggestibility, becomes even bitterly disappointed, for he was really all set to "go deep asleep," and nothing happened, not the way he expected it at all. He will be hard to get under after that, whereas, if he had been handled in an authoritarian manner, he would have responded readily to quick techniques. It takes experience to spot these subjects, and even then one can make mistakes, but this is where testing can help. Any subject whose hands lock tightly, who falls back readily, or who responds well to the eye set technique, can usually be surprised into hypnosis by transferring a test into an induction technique. If you apply a slow, permissive technique to such a subject, it will not work, or not as well as it should. On the other hand, a fast, strong approach will frequently cause resentment in the type who is not so suggestible, who may dislike such an approach, even though he wants to be hypnotized. I have found the following procedure to be the most effective and practical. I tell the patient that I am going to simply test his susceptibility. I then tell him to close his eyes and breathe very deeply, that if the three test changes are positive, he will be taken deeper.

1. Chest breathing will change to belly breathing,
2. Belly breathing will get shallow,
3. Toes will deviate.

Then he is given suggestions that these changes are occurring and then he can be taken to deeper levels for a second test. This approach is especially helpful in the event of resistance and failure, that the therapist can simply say that the patient didn't pass the test but that with a little help he would probably do very well the next time. Resistance can then be explored and resolved.

Some subjects will get the impression that if the hand levitation fails with them, that this indicates their inability to go into a deep state of hypnosis. Explain that this is not true, that each time in the future they will be able to go deeper and hand levitation is not essential. Point out that when they are ready to go deeper, the hand will rise up through their concentration—without any difficulty. The important task is to discover the true cause of the resistance and to resolve it.

REINDUCTION

Hypnotize to a light or medium trance level. Say "each time you go into hypnosis, you go deeper and deeper—deeper each time, that's the way hypnosis works—deeper each time . . . wake up now." Snap your fingers or clap your hands. Give no warning, as this would lessen the realization of the difference in the change of consciousness. Then say with authority, "deeper sleep again, deeper than ever, going deeper this time—deeper each time." Continue rapidly with deepening techniques. Each time that you awaken and reinduce the trance state, state clearly and repeatedly that, "Every time you go into hypnosis, you will go deeper. That's the way hypnosis works. Be prepared to go much deeper." Reinduction, within the same trance and at successive sessions deepens the trance. This should be explained in the beginning, and repeated from time to time, both within the trance and as a prehypnotic suggestion. The patient is in a state of heightened suggestibility just before hypnosis and immediately after hypnosis. That is the reason that particularly after hypnosis, the subject should have an opportunity to let the posthypnotic suggestions "set." Rapid awakening and reinduction can be repeated any number of times, about five or six times within the same trance. Deepening in between will break stubborn resistance markedly. The reason for this is the realization by the subject of the difference in awareness. He is compelled to admit to himself that something is happening. Not only that, but he isn't afforded the opportunity to divert his thoughts.

Another form of reinduction within the same trance is accomplished by a simple method. Say, "Now I am going to begin counting in a special way. As I count forward, you will go deeper. Presently, when I count backward, you will awaken a little more with each count backward, and then, when I resume counting forward, you will go much deeper, deeper than before. First, I will count from one to ten, and with each forward count, you will go deeper ... one ... deeper ... two ... deeper ... three ... deeper and deeper ... four ... very deep now ... five ... deeper ... deeper ... six ... deeper ... seven much deeper ... eight ... deeper ... nine ... much deeper now ... ten ... very deep ... and now, waking up a little ... nine ... a little more, eight ... waking up more, seven ... a little more, six ... more still ... five ... and NOW, going DEEPER, six, DEEPER AND DEEPER, much deeper ... seven ... deeper ... eight ... much deeper ... nine ... deeper ... ten ... very deep ... eleven ... much deeper ... twelve ... thirteen ... very deep ... fourteen ... fifteen ... sixteen ... deeper and deeper ... seventeen ... deep asleep ... eighteen ... nineteen ... twenty ... deeper asleep."

This method actually deepens the trance and brings the subject out, as the hypnotist counts backward, therefore, it is a method for deepening through reinduction within the same trance. It is effective to have the subject take up counting or counting with the hypnotist and deepening his own trance, counting forward from 20 to 30, backward to 25, awakening a little more with each backward count, and then forward to 40 or so, deepening with each count. This gives the anxious subject, the one who fears loss of control, a wonderful sense of security, when he first realizes that he can actually participate in the process of hypnotic induction. No amount of assurance that "no one can be hypnotized against his will, or that it happens because you let it happen," can compare with the awareness that he can step up or oppose the process of conditioning necessary for his therapy. This working together cooperatively and sharing control increases confidence and security feelings. This approach can be most helpful. Its greatest value is in the deepening and reawakening procedure, bringing instant realization of a change of consciousness. In this way, it heightens suggestibility.

THE NEW APPROACH—NEW TECHNIQUES

A change of scene can be often helpful. Another room, chair or couch, or soft background music—lights very low, or bright, but decidedly different from the last time, when the results were poor. If the quiet, methodical approach didn't work the last time, switch to new methods, quicker, more confusing. Take full advantage of the element of surprise. Don't repeat approaches that have failed previously. Use a different approach. If you haven't used any special effects before like lights, a hypnodisc machine, etc., do so now. My Endogenic Hypnosis Technique usually works wonderfully well with the refractory subject, and can be combined with various body-awareness techniques for pyramiding hypnosis to a deeper state. As indicated earlier, some subjects get tired and bored when gazing at exterior points of fixation.

THE AUXILIARY HYPNOTIST

(See also Miller Endogenic Technique, Chapter 4)
The testing and induction phases are conducted as usual, and at a given point, the hypnotist calls upon the auxiliary to verify the progress that is being made; sometimes no progress is evident at all, but when such a discussion in-

dicates progress, it almost invariably follows the *suggestion* that "He is going deeper, his breathing is slowing up remarkably, he's relaxing wonderfully, isn't he?" And the auxiliary confirms this in a positive voice, expressing amazement at the remarkable progress of the subject. Although the auxiliary should emphasize change, he should not grossly exaggerate. The suggestion of relaxing, and going deeper will follow, for several reasons. First, not hypnotist, but the auxiliary—usually someone with prestige —*says* his hypnosis is deepening, his breathing is more rhythmic, slower, etc. Too, this prevents the subject from thinking anything else. The exercises for induction and deepening are for this purpose, to get the subject to think *with the hypnotist*—to think the same thing that the hypnotist is thinking, *and nothing else.* When he thinks "deep asleep" to the exclusion of other thoughts, he will indeed be deep asleep.

Chapter 6

CONSIDERATIONS IN CONDUCTING
THE HYPNOTIC SESSION

Since the intellectual, critical and reasoning functions are reduced and affectivity and compliance increased in the hypnotic state, it appears logical that patients would not be able to as effectively offer resistance to analysis and would thus be better able to release repressed affect-laden conflicts.

Hypnotic transference, which can develop rapidly to a marked degree, can be effectively employed to further empathy, identification and the incorporation of feelings, thoughts, values and traits of the therapist, who in the transference fulfills a substitute parental role.

Freud believed that the peculiar susceptibility of the subject to give up control over his volition and action to the hypnotist was due to an unconscious desire on his part for libidinal gratification. Freud's co-worker, Ferenczi, recognizing the marked effects of hypnosis on the development of transference, added that hypnosis was a reactivation of the patient's infantile attitude of blind faith and implicit obedience based on both the love and fear of the parents. He further believed that the success of the hypnotist was dependent not only on the extent of transference but also upon his prestige as an all-powerful father or authority in the eyes of the patient. One can only wonder as to why Freud and his co-workers overlooked the therapeutic possibilities of utilizing hypnotic transference to speed up and facilitate the therapeutic process.

It is interesting that although Freud and many of his followers were critical of the strong authoritative approach to the patient they nevertheless incorporated the "prestige approach" in their psychoanalytic rituals. According to Freud, the analyst had to be strong and secure and inspire respect for his position. In fact, the analyst like a priest must be so strong, pure, and incorruptible as not to be susceptible to most of the mortal weaknesses of men. In addition, he should attain the acme of objectivity, but he must in the eyes of the patient be in virtually absolute authority.

ALTERATIONS IN PSYCHIC FUNCTIONS

Of particular interest are certain alterations in the psychic functions occurring in the hypnotic state. For instance, there is a marked ability to fantasize and hallucinate. As Schilder pointed out, the hypnotized subject's perceptual world is altered. He sees things others do not, and he does not see things others do. The mere command of the hypnotist can arouse new and vividly colorful images before him. This particular enhanced ability to project artistic images is beautifully exploited in the hypnography technique employed by Meares.

Similarly, following the hypnotist's command, psychosomatic effects can occur, particularly in those parts of the body which are innervated by the vegetative nervous system. Thus, by suggestion, the hypnotist can produce bodily changes which the subject could not willfully create or alter. Since affectivity, as indicated earlier, is increased in the hypnotic trance, such somatic effects occur as a result of intensified emotional reaction, i.e., vasomotor constriction or dilatation, slowing or speeding of the heart or respiration, gastrointestinal secretion and motility, diaphoresis and pupillary changes, etc. Experimentally, Forel, Schultz, Heller, and Alrutz have even elicted burn blisters by means of hypnosis. I had occasion to observe that hypnotic suggestion tended to reduce the inflammatory reaction in acute thrombophlebitis of the lower extremities. That hypnosis can influence the menstrual cycle is well known. I have found that hypnotic influence can create marked gastric nausea or emesis or can relieve these conditions when they exist. Hypnosis has been effectively employed by the author, i.e., in the successful treatment of a number of cases of pernicious vomiting in pregnancy.

The hypotonia of the hypnotic state as in the cataleptic phenomenon is a result of hypnotically induced motor cortical inhibition. In the hypnotic trance we note further that there is an accompanying marked inhibition of the cortical motor speech center with a reduction or loss of spontaneous speech. The subject will usually answer but not initiate speech. During the trance, the inhibitory effects can be partially overcome by hypnotic suggestions. The extent of the loss of voluntary motor control depends on the depth of the trance.

Of further interest is the fact that similar automatism is characteristic of certain schizophrenic states, particularly in catatonics. In the hypnotic state some degree of automatic compliance and obedience is usually manifest. A similar phenomenon is observed in the catatonic forms of dementia praecox. Patients tend to carry out instructions of others in a blind obedient manner without the exercise of critical reasoning. In the hypnotic trance, patients although compliant are capable of resisting instructions or suggestions to a limited degree, depending on the trance depth. This is particularly evident when instructions, commands or suggestions are given to the patient which he perceives as threatening or endangering his security.

In hypnosis, even though the muscle tone is very relaxed, we have noted that the tendon reflexes are responsive and in some instances even hyperreactive. This lends support to the conclusion that in this state of hypnoidal sleep the individual can be readily awakened and prepared to defend himself, if attacked.

Further support for the hypothesis that hypnosis is a form of primal sleep, is the fact that patients can be readily transferred from the hypnotized state to deep sleep. Similarly, often patients who have been trained in autohypnosis were frequently able to pass from this state into deep sleep.

ASSOCIATIVE EROTIC EXPERIENCES

The belief by some authors that hypnosis is associated with erotic experience is undoubtedly justified in certain cases. Since all affectivity is increased, it follows that sexual and erotic feelings are also accentuated. Patients with latent or overt homosexual tendencies often react to the procedure, lying on a couch or to hypnotic induction itself, with vicarious erotic feelings. In some instances, however, latent homosexuals may be quite threatened by such procedures and in such cases, in my opinion, they are not advisable. Female homosexuals may be resistive to the couch or to hypnosis. Yet, if the female patient accepts the procedure from a male therapist, it is generally therapeutically beneficial.

RELATIONSHIP INFLUENCES TRANSFERENCE

Certainly the character of the feelings transmitted depends to some degree upon the sex and personality makeup of the respective hypnotist and subject. Certainly the inner needs of humans enter into any process of communication. It has been pointed out that hysterics with a strong leaning towards dependency, devotion, and object-cathexis are most readily hypnotized, giving rise to the belief that hypnosis represents a kind of infantile submission to a strong father image. This belief is certainly supported by clinical observation. Nevertheless, it appears to be that tendencies toward autosuggestion, belief in miracles, magic, tradition, authoritarian rearing are often found in such cases and tend markedly to influence their reactions. The physician often recognizes that medication may at times represent a crutch for the patient. Similarly, any psychotherapeutic relationship utilized as a palliative for subjective relief may present the possibility of dependence rather than a realistic resolution of the patient's problem, and particularly so, if the patient is unconsciously in quest of such a dependent relationship.

Schilder noted that in compulsion-neurotics spite was dominant and that sadistic as well as masochistic anal fantasies often break through. He feels that the pleasurable submission encountered in hypnosis is related to the subject's own unconscious wish to be hurt, dominated, and overpowered. He states further that the sadist vicariously enjoys the submission of the other and the masochist the intensity of his suffering. In some cases this is undoubtedly true, however, no such general statement is clinically valid. Schilder perhaps has overlooked the fact that most patients much more frequently seek love and pleasure through submission rather than hurt.

It is important that the hypnotist not abuse the position and influence which he holds in the eyes of his subjects. For the hypnotized person, often the hypnotist has the power of a creator; he can create new things in the external world merely by his word. To be most effective therapeutically, the hypnotist must be a secure, mature, well-trained person and always have the best interests of the patient at heart. He must not misuse his powers to lead the subject to expect unrealistic miracles and magical solutions. He has no choice but to hold forth the hope of realistic goals and encourage the patient to strive earnestly for the fulfillment of his desires. To accomplish these ends, it is important that the hypnotist transfer constructive motivation, confidence, and self-acceptance to the patient. The positive transference, warm rapport and unity resulting from successful hypnotic transference greatly furthers identification with the therapist and the beneficial introjection and sharing of his feelings, wishes, counsel and mode of relating to others.

Hypnotic influence properly utilized fosters the more rapid development of positive transference, feelings of love and unity towards the therapist. The author makes strong use of positive transference and love as a therapeutic motivating factor. Love stimulates unity, togetherness and harmony as hate stimulates division, isolation and turmoil. (Miller, M. M., "The sin doctrine and the capacity to love," 2nd Int. Congress, Group Psychotherapy, Zurich 1957, *Act. Psychotherapy.*)

THE PHENOMENON OF SUGGESTION

Suggestion can be divided into two types—wakeful and hypnotic suggestion. We must differentiate between suggestion which primarily originates within the person in the form of autosuggestion and external suggestion. By means of the psychic phenomenon of suggestion, individuals can be influenced to accept beliefs, ideas, experiences or feelings, as if they were real or actually experienced by the subject. In treatment, a number of significant factors are involved which influence the process of suggestion and the ability of the patient to accept suggestion. One is the faith or trust which the patient has in the suggesting person. Another is the patient's attitude, namely, whether he is in an accepting or resistive state of mind; whether he is emotionally cooperative or resistant, whether he is attached to the suggestor or resents him; whether his mind is in an abstract or concrete state. The degree of concentration of the subject is also significant.

Such factors as the prestige and reputation of the suggestor greatly affect the suggestive process. Suggestibility, of course, is much enhanced by the authoritative and strong approach of the therapist who conveys conviction and confidence, not only verbally but through his gestures, and expression. (Repetition of the verbal suggestion enhances effect when done with proper intonation.)

Another factor is the influence of the patient's observation of other patients being hypnotized. A good example of this is in group hypnosis in which a tremendous amount of suggestive influence is generated in the group when some subjects become highly suggestible and responsive to the therapist. The augmented suggestibility of a group is similar to the herding reaction of animals in the fact of danger, etc. It is a primitive, atavistic type of collective response.

The anticipatory state of the patient is also important. A patient who anticipates a certain positive influence and effect upon himself is more likely to experience this suggestibility. Furthermore each suggestive influence which the patient experiences in himself intensifies and augments further response to suggestion. The great importance of certain symbolic gestures in enhancing the suggestibility of the patient is well expressed by Meares in his discussion of the atavistic regressive character of induction of the hypnotic state. Meares, for example, stresses that a simple suggestion is more likely to be accepted by the patient and that, as this is accepted, the patient will respond progressively to more complex suggestions.

Suggestibility can be enhanced by sedatives, anaesthetics, alcohol and drugs which sedate the ego and the reality-testing capacities. Furthermore, suggestibility can be increased by rhythmic movements, by repetitive sounds, by fatigue, and other factors. We must recognize that suggestion is not an intellectual process, but is basically an emotional one, and therefore is tremendously influenced by the affective relationship between the patient and the therapist. It is for this reason that appeals to logic, to reason, to step-by-step analysis and evaluation do not increase suggestibility but generally lessen it, because they tend to awaken the critical faculties of the mind and to activate the reality-testing capacities.

It is obvious that the faith and trust of the patient greatly enhances suggestibility. It is clear that we often believe those whom we trust without questioning. Suggestibility is enhanced when there is emotional security and absence of threat. A close relationship between the patient and therapist makes sharing of feelings and beliefs easier.

Suggestibility is increased as well when the therapist speaks in a monotone or utters monotonous repetitive sounds. We have also found experimentally that suggestibility can be greatly enhanced by exposing the patient to authoritative confirmation of the therapist's observations by others. I found that the suggestive influence could be potentiated by the utilization, as before shown, of a so-called auxiliary hypnotist technique in which one or more observers confirm the suggestions of the hypnotist. In this procedure a third person, namely, another doctor or nurse, could be used as an observer to confirm the effects occurring within the patient during initial induction.

There are a number of cultural factors which influence suggestibility. Persons who are repeatedly exposed to faith-inspiring influences, such as highly religious church goers, are often more suggestible, have a tendency to accept beliefs on faith. This applies also to some soldiers, who have become accustomed to accepting orders without question. Individuals are also more susceptible to suggestion if it is based on tribal or national ethnic customs, and they are less likely to question suggestions made by people of their own faith or cultural background than those made by representatives of unfamiliar cultures. Thus, often within a tribe the rituals and superstitions are accepted, whereas they would be completely unacceptable in another cultural framework.

Suggestibility is defined by Meares as that function of the mind which determines the acceptibility or rejection of suggestion. I would like to add that suggestibility, according to my view, is the degree to which the individual can accept impressions or suggestions without resorting to criticism, questioning, negation or to the reality-testing of these impressions.

We have mentioned some of the factors which affect suggestibility. Patients in a disturbed or threatened state of mind may be more suggestible as regards the possibility of being hurt or taken advantage of, while others may become very defensive and less suggestible. As pointed out earlier in discussing cultural factors, there is an element of selective suggestibility, for example, a mechanic would not be very receptive to suggestions concerning the repair of cars, but might be highly suggestible on the subject of religion, politics or his health. Of course, suggestibility varies greatly with the age and experience of a person in terms of reality experience and with the level of intelligence. While the level of intelligence may influence suggestibility to a point, it is an error to believe that highly intelligent people cannot be suggestible. This depends primarily on rapport between the therapist and the patient, and again on the factor of selective suggestibility, which means that people are more suggestible outside their own sphere of activity. The writer has found that often highly intelligent individuals are more suggestible when a psychophysiological approach is used on induction, with some explanation of the nature of hypnosis and the endogenic technique.

With reference to selective suggestibility, Meares points out that many patients who are inclined to be resistive to suggestions of relaxation may often be readily hypnotized by suggestions of arm levitation, and that further, many patients who resist arm levitation may be readily hypnotized by suggestions of relaxation. The therapist should carefully determine which technique to attempt. Generally the patients who are threatened by relaxation and loss of consciousness have difficulty in relinquishing conscious awareness and falling asleep. They are generally on guard and alert, and frequently tend toward compulsive behavior. With such patients, active induction procedures are generally more effective, i.e., arm levitation and rotation, etc.

As stated before, the factor of rapport is important, and patients sometimes show a selective resistance to suggestion by certain therapists, but are nonresistive to others. This was observed on a fairly large scale at our clinic where we had many young doctors training in the use of clinical hypnotic procedure. Very often the voice, attitude, expression or manner of the therapist would produce a marked resistance in the patient. Meares pointed out that suspicious paranoid persons are particularly suggestible in the area of their suspicions and paranoid projections, but are often also resistive in other areas. Certain patients are difficult to hypnotize but it is possible to exploit their suggestibility in specific areas.

Negative suggestibility is characterized by the patient's reacting in a manner opposite to the suggestion received. If it is suggested he put his left hand on his stomach, he places his right there instead. It is apparent that he is contesting and resisting the influence of the hypnotist, and is struggling against losing conscious voluntary control. He does this by opposing every suggestion in an overcompensatory manner. For example, if he is told to close the eyes, he opens them even wider. If he is told to awaken from the trance, he tries to remain in a hypnotic state. If he is told that his arm is rising, he presses it down against the couch or chair. In instances of negative suggestibility the cause of the resistance should be evaluated carefully and analyzed before any attempt is made to relax the patient. Although it is possible to hypnotize such patients, they often still remain partially resistive, and attempts to outwit their ego may incur anxiety and hostility. They can be hypnotized by exploiting their negative reactions in either of two ways. One can switch the suggestions so that if the patient does not breathe deeply the therapist suggests that the shallow breathing is an indication of good relaxation. I also use the following method, saying, "The more you try to relax, the more you will remain awake. The more you try to remain awake, the more relaxed you will become, etc." These inverted suggestions tend to confuse the negativistic patient. If these fail, other active methods may be attempted. It is often best not to proceed too energetically, but simply suggest, "You have passed the initial tests successfully and the next session you'll be able to do much better." In this manner, posthypnotic suggestion can be used to progressively deepen the trance.

In the hypnotic state we observe such basic changes as alterations of the psychic functions, dissociation, regression, hypersuggestibility, hypermnesia, hyperaffectivity, some degree of dissociation which may be made more selective with selective concentration, lifting of repression, increased rapport, and altered transference responses. This regression may be spontaneous or gradual in character. Due to the lifting of repression, hysterical, compulsive-obsessive and regressive behavior may become manifest as well as emotional catharsis and abreaction. An increased tendency toward fantasy and hallucination can occur, and can be either spontaneous or gradual in character. Patients may show some tendency toward histrionics and mimicry and, as Meares points out, may behave in a manner in which they believe a hypnotized person behaves. Also, in the hypnotic state patients often have the capacity to communicate more freely and to feel more deeply due to the lifting of repressions.

Posthypnotic manifestations may be amnesia, or behavior inspired by posthypnotic suggestion. We may have posthypnotic sleep which may be spontaneous or gradual in onset. Posthypnotic execution of commands or instruction is a result of motivation planted in the unconscious. When giving posthypnotic suggestion, it is best to word the suggestions in such a manner as to express the wish, intent, or objective of the subject, i.e., "You will avoid sickening sweets, starchy and fatty foods because you want to become slender, attractive and healthy."

THE HYPNOTIC INTERVIEW

After the patient is sufficiently relaxed and in a reasonably receptive and compliant state, the hypnotic interview can begin. It is suggested to the patient that he will feel more like talking about his feelings and thoughts, that it will make him feel more relaxed and happier to express his feelings, that words will flow like a brook, clear, continuously and that he will be able to discharge the tensions he feels more freely. He will be told that when he is asked questions he will try to answer them and express what he really feels. He will be asked if there is any one person or situation on his mind, appropriate questions such as whom he feels angry at or whom he misses most, what is his greatest concern, etc. Under hypnosis the patient is better able to respond to specific questions. Feeling memories are enhanced under hypnosis. The patient can more readily relate what or whom he fears most. If asked broad questions, such as, "What are you afraid of?" there may be hesitation and sometimes no response, for the patient may fear many things. A question such as, "Who hurt you the most?" or "What happened that was the most painful memory in school? may be asked. Major traumas are usually better retained and communicated under hypnosis. Specific directives, guidelines and questions are helpful to the patient in the hypnotic state.

MANNER OF COMMUNICATING DURING THE TRANCE

The hypnotist must in the eyes of the patient present a strong, secure, authoritative image. He must not be hesitant, wavering, hurried, stammering or inarticulate. He should speak in a strong, confident, clear voice. Although authoritative, he should not be unreasonable and make excessive demands or ignore the needs of the patient. Rather, he should qualify his suggestions and instructions by stating, i.e., to his female patient seeking to lose weight, "You desire so much to be attractive, healthy and happy so you will participate in your favorite forms of physical recreation because it will bring you the joy you seek and benefit you both physically and mentally. You will carry out my instructions because that will help you to become attractive and healthy." It is best to always align the aims of the hypnotist with those of the patient.

Thus, one can strengthen positive motivations and desires of the patient. It is best not to overstate or exaggerate. If the patient cannot become a beauty, it would be best to use the word "prettier" or "more attractive," rather than to say, "You will become beautiful;" overexaggeration can be harmful and disillusioning, particularly if the patient cannot attain the image set for her. It is therefore best to set realistic goals.

In conducting a hypnotic session, the hypnotist must be most careful not to say anything that might excite undue anxiety in the patient. Patients under hypnosis often tend to be much more impressionable and tend more toward obsessive and phobic fixations.

It is always best, as a rule of thumb, to utilize a positive approach, i.e., "You will feel wonderful, refreshed, happier, etc." In conducting the hypnotic session, it is always better to permit the patient to express his feelings. Questioning as regards their feelings, thoughts, and experiences in a kindly, sympathetic manner can be quite productive. Trying to provoke a response by making assertions may be hazardous, traumatic, and counter productive.

A leading question like the following may be revealing, "Have you ever been hurt badly by anyone as a child—your mother?—father?—brothers?—sisters?—a teacher?" The patient may begin to describe a painful episode. "Tell me more about it." A follow-up question could be, "Has anyone ever hurt you like that more recently?"

Deja Senti: Helping the patient to feel and relive what he has felt before. An illustration is if the patient says, "I feel so unsure of myself, so afraid I'll fail," the therapist can ask, "I wonder when you first felt like that before." The patient, at this point, can be regressed:

Therapist: "You will now go back through teenage, adolescence, preadolescence, back until the time when you first felt like that, when it first happened. You'll tell me how it first happened."

Patient: "It was in the fifth grade. There was that Mrs. M. She hurt my feelings badly. She bawled me out and punished me right in front of the whole class. What hurt worse she humiliated me in front of people I really cared for and wanted to make a good impression on like that girl Carol I liked so much. That really hurt!"

Therapist: "Didn't anyone ever hurt you like that before?"

Patient: "I remember that Mom bawled me out pretty badly when I was eight for wetting the bed. She said she was going to tell my friends if I didn't stop. I felt so upset, so ashamed when she told them. That's something I've never gotten over. I hated her for doing that to me. I couldn't stand being laughed at, made a fool of, shamed."

Therapist: "How did it make you feel about yourself?

Patient: "Frankly, it made me feel like 'shit.' "

Upon termination of the session conducted in hypnotic regression, the patient can be told that he is coming back through the years, through preadolescence, adolescence and as he comes into the present to try to recall feelings of hurt reoccurring that were like the feelings he had had when mother had shamed him so badly.

In this manner earlier feelings and experiences can be tied into more recent experiences.

TECHNIQUE FOR HANDLING AGE REGRESSION

There are two aims in age regression under hypnosis; to facilitate memory and recollection of past traumatic events and earlier feelings, the other to effect revivification, whereby the subject may relive and recall earlier experiences with the original emotional impact. It is difficult to induce a satisfactory regression when the patient is in an insufficiently deep trance. Loss of time sense occurs best in a medium to deep trance. Regression in the hypnotic state is greatly facilitated by the loss of time sense of the hypnotized subject. Regression, on the whole, is a safe procedure providing that the hypnotherapist is properly trained in psychotherapy and is capable of properly assessing the patient's ego strength and capacity to handle emotionally traumatic material. Furthermore, the therapist should possess sufficient insight and awareness so that he can quickly observe any untoward disturbances within the patient, i.e., manifestations of acute anxiety, hysterical conversion symptoms, etc. Prior to hypnotic regression, adequate information concerning the patient's background and history can be most helpful. Considerable attention should be given to the question of whether this patient has had any previous psychiatric history, mental breakdown or psychotic reactions, if possible, by means of hypnotic regression to explore the root causes of their difficulties.

Generally, the beneficial catharsis resulting from the emotional reliving of earlier repressed conflicts and trauma, with the consequent release of tension results in a general improvement of the patient's condition. Following emergence from the trance, it is usually therapeutic to consciously ventilate and discuss material derived during the session. Again, the therapist must be guided by his appraisal of the patient's condition as to whether he is yet able to confront such disturbing revelations. If the patient's condition reveals deeper disturbance and where insight is limited, it is wise to proceed slowly in conveying any traumatic material to the patient. Often, in such instances, a gradual multistage approach is better, both from the point of view of lessening trauma as well as in building insight. Often by repeated exposure to traumatic episodes, the patient may become desensitized and freed of his fear, guilt, etc.

It is good when attempting regression that the therapist have a favorable rapport with the patient. The subject should feel that his interests are the primary concern of the hypnotist. His faith in the therapist greatly lessens his anxiety and he is more likely to feel safe and protected and to anticipate benefit.

With reference to the induction of age regression, it is best at first not to proceed too energetically in inducing regression. If the subject tends to develop marked affective, hysterical or disturbed reactions, it is best not to regress the patient further and the patient should be brought out of the trance. After the patient is pacified, it is advisable to attempt, whenever possible, to uncover the cause of the disturbing reaction. Prior to induction, it is helpful to have the subject record a number of projections such as writing his name, drawing an image of self, or his parents or other objects for purposes of comparative analysis afterwards.

The following procedure as employed by J. Slone, is recommended following induction: regress the subject slowly to the day before, the week and month before, a year ago, two years, three years, going back in time gradually. It is good to give the subject sufficient time for the surroundings and impressions to "set." For instance, if the subject is 25 years old and it is desired to regress him to the age of seven, he should be taken back to 24, 23, 20, 18, 15, 12, nine, etc. In this manner, he is permitted enough time in each phase of the regression to experience impressions and recollections. The production of such material depends usually to a large degree on the affective state of the patient. It is the reexperiencing of former hurt feelings that facilitate recollection of past painful events *(Deja senti)*.

These recollections may become very vivid as the past becomes the present. Often one can observe the voice changing as the regression progresses as though the patient is acting out the behavior of a younger person representing an earlier level of his life. One can, for instance, mention a significant event, a birthday, Christmas, graduation, beginning school, or some specific occasion and have the subject relate where he is, what he is doing, how he feels on this occasion, etc. If the trance is sufficiently deep and the subject is permitted adequate time, he may actually reexperience the event and upon suggestion speak as though he were at the regressed age as though it were in the present. If after suggestions that he is now at school age and he talks readily about his school friends, his teacher, his pets, etc., but says, "I was there in school" rather than "I am there in school now," he is not fully regressed. It is then necessary to suggest, "You will feel like you are there in school now." If he mentions a teacher's name, as well as other names, events or places, he is regressed. If he says, "I am at school, in the first grade and my teacher's name —then exclaims, "She is teaching us!" then his regression represents a true regression. Should he be successfully regressed back prior to the time of speech, he will be unable to speak, but may make infantile noises and cry and laugh like a baby. Generally, a nonverbal signal should be preestablished with the subject, just in case he suddenly ceases to speak. The subject is told that if he is tapped on the head or shoulder, he will be enabled to speak again. Slone points out that persons in a true regression who did not speak English until at a certain age may often start speaking in a foreign tongue at the age prior to speaking English. At this point, they will not usually respond when spoken to in English. It is here that the nonverbal signal can be employed and a touch on the head is then usually sufficient to bring the subject back to the English-speaking age.

Some subjects, when regressed, appear to be just acting or simulating. They tend to role play and act out what they think the behavior was at a specific time. They may reveal a combination of both role playing and revivification.

The character of the regression that is achieved is primarily based on the depth of the trance and how effectively the suggestions are given, particularly with regard to how strongly fixated they are in the subject's mind and the extent to which they are accepted; that is, the degree of resistance. One must remember that the regressed patient's mind usually works slowly and he waits for the anticipated next suggestion from the hypnotist. In a sense, the hypnotist is like a person playing a victrola. With each suggestion, he selects and initiates the playing off of another record in the patient's mind.

The subject may often, during the regressed state, transfer to the therapist as though he were a father, a mother, an uncle, an aunt, a brother, a sister, teacher or friend. He has apparently lost a finer sense of discriminating identities, reacting in a more infantile, indiscriminate manner.

At times, when a subject is regressed to the particular age when he suffered a traumatic incident, he may block. He may manifest resistance by spontaneously awakening from the trance and resisting being hypnotized again, or he may remain in the trance and resist further regression. Subconsciously, he does not wish to reexperience the painful episode. Generally, this can be best handled indirectly by regressing the patient to a time not too remote from the incident and gradually permitting him to reveal the traumatic experience. In order to reduce resistance, it is good to reassure the subject that whatever is being done is being done for his benefit and that as a result of facing these painful episodes, he can soon anticipate the rewards of happiness and peace of mind and that the more he cooperates, the sooner he will achieve relief.

A highly interesting case was the following: Bill, a 33-year old, married man was suffering from deep anxieties. When he was alone his anxieties became more intense. His fear pervaded all through his life. He felt insecure about his marriage, his sexual life, his job, etc. He manifested a marked fear of physical injury. He was unable to explain the source of his persistent anxiety.

Bill was hypnotized and regressed in stages rather rapidly through the 20's, the teens, adolescence—preadolescence. It was suggested he would go back, back until he could recall the first most fearful experience in his life. As he regressed back to an early childhood level, he was suddenly seized with an excruciating pain in the calf of his right leg. At that point he was feeling increasing pain and appeared to shrink with a terrified expression on his face. "Bill," I asked, "Who is hurting you so—What's happening?" Then he remembered and exclaimed, "It's that big white rooster which is picking at my right leg and tearing my flesh. It's bleeding. I'm screaming helplessly for my mother, but she is not around. I am terror stricken." The incident, as was recalled in the waking state occurred when Bill was three and a half. It was on a Missouri farm. His father had left his mother. She had no one to leave him with and had to go to town. So she put him in the chicken yard so he couldn't wander off. Bill showed a remarkable reduction in anxiety after the painful traumatic episode was abreacted and discussed. Of interest was the fact that Bill experienced the pain before he could recall the episode itself.

Communications of a traumatic character can often be achieved through the technique of automatic writing. Automatic writing is direct, rapid, less painful, very revealing and can be effective at a lesser degree of trance depth than with verbal communication. The author has employed this procedure with some degree of success. On the whole, however, with the exception of patients who tend to block verbally, it is best to attempt to retain verbal communication since it is productive in a higher percentage of cases. It is easier with verbal communication to obtain a greater amount of associated and background material. Automatic writing can certainly be most useful in specific cases of severe trauma and in which resistance to verbal communication is evident. The central conflicts thus revealed can later, at an appropriate time for the patient, be consciously ventilated and discussed with therapeutic benefit.

CASE EXAMPLES OF CLINICAL APPLICATION OF REGRESSION

Case A. John, a 32-year old engineer was found to be depressed, anxious, socially passive and withdrawn, and had for some years been suffering from partial impotence. John was married and for one year previously his wife was confined to a mental hospital suffering a manic-depressive psychosis. John had marked difficulty in communicating, particularly regarding his own personal problems and it was therefore decided to employ hypnosis. He was hypnotized without difficulty. Following several sessions during which his trance was progressively deepened, the first attempt to regress was made. He was gradually regressed back through the twenties, the teens, adolescence and preadolescence and then to early childhood. His early life centered on primarily two persons, his mother and an older brother, Bill. He described how stern, strict and severe they were with him and his dread of both. His mother, a widow, had literally given his older brother, Bill, a carte blanche as far as exercising authority over John was concerned. Bill often punished him sometimes severely even for trivialities. He appeared to enjoy dominating and hurting his younger brother. His mother, a nurse, was often away and consequently John was largely at Bill's mercy. John became increasingly timid, docile and inhibited. This was apparent in his first conference with me. He was utterly lacking in spontaneity. During the third session while regressed, John recalled a scene in bed with his mother when he was about three years of age. He was lying alongside of her and felt a desire to touch one of her breasts but was unable to do so. He felt possessed by a fear, a feeling that this was forbidden. He spoke at length about his stern, religious mother who literally tabooed any mention of sex or reproduction and conveyed the impression to him that she considered the naked human body as utterly sinful, lustful, vulgar and despicable. Although he recalled, on the other

hand, moments when his calvinistic mother managed repeatedly to leave the bathroom door ajar while she was
unclad and when on such occasions he or his brothers
dared to peek and satisfy their erotic curiosity, they were
almost always reprimanded and made to feel guilty. John
was then progressed from his early regressed childhood
state to his wedding night when he was 23. He was in bed
with Mary, his newly wed, and attempted to touch her
breasts, but once again was seized by the same anxiety and
felt unable to. When questioned further, it became increasingly clear how Mary in her hunger for demonstrative love
and affection was eventually forced more and more to assume an aggressive role. He went on to relate how his
passivity continued to increasingly disturb Mary and how
she began to develop alternate states of agitation and depression, finally culminating in a manic-depressive psychosis.

As a result of these disclosures, it was possible to assist
John in obtaining sufficient insight into his personality
problems. The communications were consciously discussed and evaluated, his disturbed feelings ventilated and
for the first time, John could recognize the absurdity and
infantile nature of his attitude toward marriage and sexual
life. He was now able to see how he had literally driven
Mary to a mental breakdown. Shortly afterwards, his impotence diminished completely, and as a result of his own
improvement, he was able to play an important part in
helping his wife back to mental health and happiness.

Case B. Ralph, 29-years old, a newspaper man, revealed bisexual tendencies and impotence towards the opposite sex. After four sessions in which he was put
repeatedly into successively deeper trances and regressed,
he was able to recall and affectively reexperience an episode in which his mother, who was divorced from his father, attempted to seduce him when he was but eight years

old. He described in detail how she had him straddle her nude body, fondled his penis and then placed his penis at the vaginal orifice. He recalled vividly the erotic pleasure which he experienced. He recalled feeling guilty and disturbed afterward. Ralph later disclosed under hypnosis how he felt erotically aroused by older women who showed him demonstrative affection and caressed him. It was further confirmed that he developed such guilt reactions as a result that he had unconsciously tended to repress all normal sexual feelings towards the opposite sex and turned toward engaging in erotic pleasures with boys and men, i.e., mutual masturbation, sodomy and fellatio. Under hypnosis, he revealed that he felt more comfortable with male sexual partners. He also revealed evidence of growing self-contempt, guilt and some self-destructive impulses. As a result of hypnotherapy and group therapy, Ralph was soon enabled to resolve his incestuous guilt and blocks toward the opposite sex. His inner conflicts were consciously ventilated and discussed. As a result, he was able to resolve the homosexuality and to develop normal feelings of attachment to a woman, which culminated in marriage.

Case C. An interesting case of hypnotic regression was that of a 32-year old woman who was suffering from obesity and depression. A psychologist, she could not understand the reasons for her compulsive eating. She was regressed back through the 20's, teenage, adolescence, preadolescence, back to three years of age. She had been given the suggestion that she would recall an early upsetting episode. She recalled that the cat had had kittens. She asked, "Mommy, if the mother cat dies, what will happen to the kittens?" Her mother replied, "Then the kittens will die." So food became equated with staying alive. This explained a great deal to this patient who was capable of excellent insight as a result of her becoming aware of the cause of her eating compulsion. Her overeating has ceased.

USE OF REGRESSION TECHNIQUE IN FORENSIC PSYCHIATRY

I have found the hypnotic-regression technique quite useful in forensic psychiatry. It is often possible, particularly with youthful offenders, to help them relive a criminal act. One can elicit a vivid description not only of the act itself, but of the background influences, motives, and circumstances involved. Often, subjects reveal where stolen loot and weapons were concealed. Hypnotic regression may also be employed as in the following instance in which the most important prosecution witness in a murder trial was unable to recall the type and color of a car in which the murderer had made his getaway three years earlier. The witness was regressed back to the original time and scene of the crime and was then able to describe the color and make of the car. It is most important in such instances not to offer suggestions but rather have the subject recall the details and circumstances and convey his own impressions.

SOME SPECIAL HYPNOTHERAPEUTIC TECHNIQUES

Placebos and Medication

The placebo is sometimes given to a patient in the form of pills or placebo solutions to enhance suggestion, etc. Obviously, these have no real curative value, usually, except in the patient's mind. A placebo can actually be given, with the suggestion that it will cause the subject to go into a deep trance. The effects of medication such as tonics, hormones, and vitamins used as placebos can be enhanced by suggestion that it will cause the subject to go into a deep trance. Pressures and passes are used much the same way —they work because the subject thinks they do. Various "hypnotic areas" can be pressed, with suggestions like this: "As I press on your hypnotic centers, the temples, you will feel yourself going deeper—pressing on these areas causes you to go much deeper." The temples and back of the neck are suggestible points for pressure. A cooling liquid can be sprayed on the back of the neck, giving a cool feeling, at the same time giving suggestions that this is a form of hypnotizing anaesthetic which will take them deeper into the trance.

Narcohypnosis

Narcohypnosis should, in my opinion, only be employed when the patient is completely resistive to frank hypnosis and there is no other alternative. Various drugs are used to produce hypnosis, the most commonly used ones being sodium amythol and sodium pentothal. These two drugs act quickly and leave no prolonged hangover. The drug is injected into the median basilic vein in the antecubital fossa. Dosage will vary, three to about fourteen grains in distilled water, 10 cc or more. As the patient counts backward from one hundred, he becomes less and less audible. As the voice of the patient becomes quite low, it is best to halt the injection. Too much of the drug will induce sleep and make the interview impossible. When the patient stops counting, the jaw drops, relaxation is noticeable, hypnotic suggestion will produce a proper hypnotic state in some subjects, but not all. They will probably to to sleep before the suggestions can become effective, have a good sleep, and remember nothing. It is best to inject too little than too much. More can be administered if necessary. When they go into narcohypnosis, the hypnotist may suggest that hereafter the subject will enter a deep hypnotic trance without drugs, any time that the hypnotist gives the instruction. A curious fact is that most subjects will swear that they were not hypnotized, just "knocked out," that the whole thing was a failure. But if they are induced later (a few minutes to a few hours), they will usually immediately go into a deep trance and be quite compliant. It seems amazing that so few people who use drugs have tried this technique. It works extremely well. The real value of drugs lies in the proper afteruse of the subject's state of mind. If the dosage is administered too rapidly, it is useless, because the patient only loses consciousness. It is not the hypnotic condition which helps the patient, but what happens under it and after it. I do not use narco-hypnosis often because such drugs tend to diminish rather than to increase the capacity to communicate, while frank hypnosis does not cause any cortical depression or inhibition.

By Example

It is a known fact that some people are much more suggestible after witnessing a hypnosis demonstration. Seeing someone else "go under" can influence a subject very strongly. This is providing the demonstration is a pleasant and enjoyable experience for the subject. The stage hypnotist always relies on this factor, selecting very suggestible subjects to demonstrate on first, and in doing this, prepares others for quicker induction. When you have a difficult subject, let him witness someone else being hypnotized, as though it was accidental. Better yet, put him in group hypnotic sessions. When he sees the other members of the group making progress with hypnosis, and through hypnosis, he is more likely to lose his reluctance to being hypnotized. Often a subject who hasn't reached a medium trance state after several sessions will go into a deep trance during the very first group session. The best approach is to have several in the group report on their progress during the past week, i.e., how the posthypnotic suggestions and self-hypnosis or other phases of the work are progressing. Then, take a good subject and demonstrate, putting him under, giving suggestions, or produce automatic writing or drawing, and posthypnotic suggestion. Everyone likes to "do well," and reports of positive results from hypnotic suggestions will encourage the slow subject. He will begin to get the idea that if others can accomplish this, so can he. Aside from a change of attitude on a conscious level, the observer is actually more suggestible after being in an actual hypnotic situation in which he observes positive results.

Group Hypnosis

Group hypnosis can be very useful as an adjunctive to group therapy. It also makes possible the speeding up of the development of transference, recovery of blocked feelings and memories and furthering of discharges of feelings in the group. From point of view of economics effective group therapy makes psychotherapy less of an economic burden to the underprivileged.

The phenomena of "synpulsion," described by the author, involving the potentiation of collective feeling and group interaction can be constructively exploited in group hypnosis. Group hypnosis lends itself well for hypnoaversion treatment, i.e., for smokers, alcoholics, drug addicts, and obese patients. Group hypnotherapy is facilitated by treating a common problem in a group. If one alcoholic vomits while in the trance, others in the group under hypnosis may respond strongly and often readily respond to suggestions of nausea and vomiting upon the smell or taste of alcoholic beverages. The dread and aversion increases markedly as they perceive the misery of their fellow patient.

Posthypnotic suggestion given in a group can be quite motivating and productive, particularly in breaking down initial barriers to communication. Those most affected by the suggestions given can activate those who are more resistive.

Group hypnosis is no more difficult than individual hypnosis, and it might well become the most effective technique for accelerating therapy, for handling juvenile delinquency, alcoholism, drug addiction, and a practical measure for preventing mental illness. Group therapy has the advantages of easing a too heavy case load, lowering cost, and providing a spirit of cooperation. Difficult subjects, or those requiring special handling, such as drug addicts and alcoholics will benefit further through individual therapy. However, in employing group hypnosis, it is best to carefully select those patients who desire to be in a group and are cooperative. Unccoperative, refractory patients can be quite disturbing and counterproductive in group hypnotherapy.

Chapter 7

HYPNOTHERAPY AND PSYCHOTHERAPY

Differential Diagnosis and Treatment of Functional Disorders

Hypnosis can be an invaluable aid in differential diagnosis. It is of particular value in distinguishing hysterical conditions from organic illness, as for example, in hysterical blindness or paralysis. I recall the case of a middle-aged woman who was in an acute state of anxiety because she had gone to her physician complaining of an inability to swallow food. The physician had sent her to a leading chest surgeon who stated that she had an oesophageal obstruction. He told her that only surgery could correct the condition; however, he added that the mortality rate in mediastinal surgery was very high. In a panic and in desperation the patient had contacted me. After she was hypnotized, she was given suggestions that she would swallow very easily and was offered some warm milk which she had no difficulty swallowing. After two sessions in which it became quite clear that her condition was psychogenic, the patient was in such excellent shape that she cancelled her third visit exclaiming that she could now "swallow the Queen Mary."

Another case was that of a 12-year old boy at a correctional school, who, upon hearing of his grandmother's death, became extremely depressed, fearful and complained of being blind. The lad was hypnotized and upon suggestion was able to see without difficulty. With tears, he related that his grandmother had raised him and he felt completely helpless and lost as a result of her death.

Another case was that of an 18-year old male athlete who complained of a left half side paralysis, his left arm and leg were immobilized and limp. After being hypnotized, he was able to move both his left hand and left leg without difficulty. When asked why he had gotten so terribly emotionally upset, he became tearful and explained that he had no one in the world but his grandmother who had raised him and that she had just recently suffered a stroke. He had repressed his fears and developed hysterical conversion symtoms. It was interesting that he had incorporated his grandmother's paralysis and had become afflicted on the same side, namely, the left side of the body.

Another case was that of a 42-year old woman, mother of seven children who had been lying in a local hospital for nine months claiming that she was paralyzed in both legs. She had become quite a nursing problem to the hospital. I succeeded in hypnotizing her without difficulty. I had the head of the bed elevated so that the limbs were hanging down slightly. There was marked muscular disuse atrophy of both legs. I then pushed the right leg upward and gave her suggestions that she would be able to move her right leg and push my hand down. Of course, her right leg fell because of gravity pushing my lightly resisting hand downward and then I remarked, "Mary, it is amazing, your right leg is moving, and now you are going to move your left leg." I did similarly with the left leg. I then gave her suggestions that she would move her feet. Then strong suggestions were given that she was getting stronger and stronger and that she now would begin to push the walker and follow it, that she would be doing this because she wanted to be able to walk for the sake of her children and that she now knew that she could move her legs but that she would have to practice and exercise her legs. To the amazement of members of the hospital staff who were observing, she pushed the walker into the corridor, slowly following it and was walking down the corridor precisely when her husband was coming up to visit her. He was absolutely dumbfounded, ran up to her, and embraced her crying, "Mary, you're walking," whereupon she awakened from the trance. Soon afterwards with the help of physiotherapy and exercise, plus additional hypnotic suggestions, Mary regained the full use of her legs.

The following case illustrates my procedure for treating hysterical paralysis. The patient, a 24-year old prisoner, was complaining of a progressive paralysis of his left hand and arm over a two-year period. A prison physician referred the case to a neurologist who according to the patient, told him that there was nothing he could do for him. Undoubtedly, the neurologist recognized the condition as hysteria but was unable to help the patient to resolve his condition.

The patient was hypnotized without difficulty. I then gave strong suggestions that he would put his unaffected hand on his left hand and that then he would be able to put his left hand on his right. He complied without difficulty. I then suggested that he could and would open and close his fist which he complied with. I subsequently challenged him by commanding, "You will now open your eyes and see your left hand moving." As he did, I then said, "You are not paralyzed. You have excellent function in your left hand and arm. Since his symptoms began about two years earlier,

I asked, "What happened just before your arm became affected two years ago?" He became very emotional, tears began to flow and in a choked-up voice he said, "My foster mother, the only one that ever loved me was dying of cancer." I then asked whether she had any impairment of her arms or legs and in a low voice he said, "Yes," it was her left arm and hand that she couldn't move for some months prior to her death. My patient had obviously incorporated her symptoms. All of this was consciously ventilated with the patient. He admitted that he had used the paralysis as an emotional crutch for secondary gain to obtain sympathy and concern and protection. Today, after nine months, he still had not had a return of his symptoms. He was given follow-up group psychotherapy.

Hypnotherapy has proven to be of great value in the treatment of speech problems. Stammering and stuttering are functional disorders and represent often deep-seated neurotic defenses which have become established generally early in life. Under hypnosis, these defense mechanisms can be explored and the etiology usually uncovered. Patient investigation is important in such instances. Hypnotic and posthypnotic suggestion can be given to facilitate speech retraining. An example of this was that of a 19-year old college student who stuttered since about four to five years of age. Under hypnosis he revealed that he had early developed marked apprehension of his father who was of a rather explosive, violent temperament. He had discovered early also that if his voice trembled or if he stammered, his father wasn't as harsh with him. His speech problem also caused his mother to act more protective of him vis-a-vis his father. He had never dared confront his father. He was given strong posthypnotic suggestions that when his father came to my office with him, he would for the first time really tell him what he thought of his past harshness and cruelty, and he would verbally vent his strongly repressed cumulative rage. He did this in a dramatic fashion to an astonished father. His speech problem resolved rapidly after that session.

THE TREATMENT OF PERSONALITY DISORDERS

Through experience I have found that hypnosis is of remarkable value in personality modification. One summer I treated a fishing captain on an island off the coast for alcoholism by my hypnoaversion method. The treatment was successful to the extent that the patient J. was rapidly conditioned so that he became nauseated and vomited every time he smelled an alcoholic beverage, reliving his worst hangover symptoms. Since I had to leave to return to Washington, I was concerned about who would give J. the follow-up treatments. Since he and his wife desired privacy, I decided that I would show his wife how to give the treatments. Five days later I received a distress call from the wife informing me that the treatment was working fine except that although J. vomited when he smelled or tasted liquor, he nevertheless kept on drinking and vomiting as though he were determined to sabotage the treatment. I went back to see him soon after and found him intoxicated. After dunking him in the ocean and plying him with black coffee, we were able to communicate about his feelings and hurts, past and present. He discussed his overpowering, dominant mother, his passive, weak father who drank excessively. I then realized my error. I had given his aggressive, dominant wife the power to emasculate J. even more. Since there was the future welfare of six children to be considered, I had to think of an alternative approach. Suddenly it occurred to me that I should, if possible, try to do the opposite. After some persuasion, I convinced the wife to submit to hypnosis. I hypnotized her and then after instructing J. how to, I transferred the power to hypnotize his wife to him. J. was a bit apprehensive at first, to be sure, since he had never been in control and had always submitted. This was an entirely new role for him. He did and interestingly, J. who had been suffering from impotence, developed an erection while he was hypnotizing his wife. After he completed the induction and had given her the specified suggestions to enhance her femininity and to improve their relationship, he awakened her. He promptly took her into a bedroom and then had very gratifying coitus for the first time in months. J. came out looking remarkably different. When I asked J. how he felt he remarked, "Wonderful." I then asked if he'd like a drink. He answered quickly, "I don't need one. If I continue to feel like this, "I'll never need one."

THE TREATMENT OF PHOBIAS BY HYPNOTIC DESENSITIZATION

In 1959 I published a report on the use of a specific type of hypnotic aversion therapy (see Chapter nine) which I had developed for the treatment of alcoholism. Since then I have applied this treatment with considerable success and adapted it to the treatment of nicotinism, obesity, sex problems, and phobias.

The rationale was the ability of the patient under hypnosis to relive a formerly revolting experience (hangover, nausea) upon the smell or taste of alcoholic spirits. This phenomenon I have termed *Deja Senti,* the ability to regress back and relive, revivify, feel a traumatic experience that happened earlier as though it were happening again. The patient was then systematically conditioned by means of hypnotic suggestion to become progressively more revolted by the smell or taste of alcoholic spirits.

If sensitization to a past traumatic or unpleasant experience can be intensified by means of hypnotic suggestion, is it not reasonable to assume that by the same means such traumas might be desensitized? And in this way, the patient with a phobic or disgust reaction could be repeatedly confronted with the dreaded situation and the disturbing reaction reduced and finally eliminated. In fact, confronting once fearful situations can even be made pleasurable.

Clinical experience over a longer period using hypnosis in the manner described here indicates that it is possible to eliminate phobias as well as such unhealthy habits as excessive smoking and drinking and obesity. This explains the technique I have developed and describes several cases which represent a variety of phobic reactions treated in this manner.

It has been my experience that when the phobic situation is recreated in the hypnotic state, the individual reacts with acute anxiety. The depth of his reaction can serve as a general indication not only of the depth of the hypnotic induction, but also of the depth of the trauma. Under hypnosis, the patient faces the dreaded experience in all its awesome reality. But the dreaded climax (death, disfigurement, pain, injury) does not occur. As a result, considerable apprehension is lost. Each time the confrontation takes place and nothing morbid results, underlying anxiety is diminshed. It is suggested that "nothing has occurred and that nothing will occur." Furthermore, when he is told that he had handled himself very well under the trying circumstances involved in the fear situation, apprehension and attendant anxiety generally rapidly disappear.

This reliving of traumatic circumstances under hypnosis has been used successfully on a variety of phobias, the major ones being acrophobia, a fear of heights and driving over bridges, of death, of assault or injury, claustrophobia (enclosed places or being smothered), aquaphobia and dread of air travel. The technique employed by the author is the Miller method of hypnotic induction which was first presented by him at the Fourth International Conference on Psychotherapy. (Endogenic hypnosis: Simpler and more

effective procedure for hypnotic induction and prolongation, *Amer. J. Soc. Psychiat.* 1:24–30 Autumn 1959.) The
following case histories further illustrate the hypnotherapeutic technique involved:

Case 1: A 39-year old woman complained that she was
unable to drive over bridges. Whenever she approached a
bridge she was seized by panic, felt virtually paralyzed, and
was unable to proceed onto and across the bridge without
great anxiety. This was a very real problem for her because
she had to drive over bridges in order to go to and from
work.

She was put into a medium depth trance and told she
was behind the wheel of her car, driving casually down the
road on a pleasant summer day. Further, she was going to
drive over the highest bridge in the world, several thousand
feet above the water. She was given suggestions to stay in
her lane, drive across the bridge, then turn off on the clo-
verleaf across the bridge and return again over the same
bridge. She was complimented on her driving and on the
control and composure she exhibited throughout this obviously trying experience. She was noticeably less apprehensive crossing the fantasied bridge the second time. Again
the instructive suggestions were repeated and she was complimented, reinforcing her gradually emerging self-confidence and building positive affect.

She was then told to turn her car around and cross and
recross the bridge again. It was suggested that she would
feel less anxiety each time and that she would begin to
enjoy the experience increasingly. Furthermore, she was
told that she would feel increasingly calm and relaxed while
driving. The anxiety reducing compliments and suggestions were repeated each time she drove across the imagi-
nary bridge. It was suggested that on the fifth time across,
she would feel so happy that she would sing. On the fifth
crossing she began to hum, then sing to herself. The sixth

time she felt no apprehension whatever. Her mood was that of elation.

During the week which followed her hypnotherapy, this patient felt a strong compelling need to test her feelings, and she drove over virtually every bridge in the Washington area, including the Chesapeake Bay Bridge near Annapolis. It has been 18 months since her hypnotherapy and her fear of bridges has never returned.

Case 2. This was an attractive 21-year old woman in the process of separating from her husband. She manifested marked fear of being assaulted, especially at night. She therefore remained at home in the evenings, with a German shepherd watchdog at her side. She would not leave the house after dark.

Under hypnosis she revealed the following incident. Several months prior to her separation, her husband and a friend played a sadistic joke on her. As she returned home from work one evening, they sprang at her from the bushes as if to attack her. She was terrified and fled. Under hypnosis she was made to relive the experience. However, it was suggested that she would realize that it was all a ridiculous joke. In this way her anxiety was diminished. She was made to reexperience the incident again with the suggestion that the joke would be at the perpetrators. It was suggested she would not only feel less tense but would, in fact, laugh at the whole situation. After reliving the experience several times, she felt no anxiety whatever and treated the incident as absurd. Follow-up of the case six months later revealed that the phobia had completely vanished.

Case 3. This was the case of a 30-year old woman who was afraid to travel by airplane. Under hypnosis she was taken on repeated flights on a fantasied vacation trip. She went through the whole experience, from check-in to seating on the plane, take-off, the flight itself, with some mild turbulence, and a smooth landing. It was suggested that on each flight she would feel more and more secure, and enjoy the flight to a greater and greater degree. After several hypnotic sessions this patient joyously anticipated air travel. She then went to a travel agency and booked a vacation flight to Jamaica. Prior to the actual flight she came in for another treatment. She enjoyed not only the hypnotic fantasied flight to and from Jamaica, but the actual flight as well. Since hypnotherapy, she collects travel literature and plans trips to visit friends and family and next year's vacation, all of which involve air travel.

The basis for this patient's fear of flying was discovered during hypnotherapy. She had a weak and undemonstrative father with a violent temper. Her mother was domineering and aggressive. The patient related to her husband in much the same manner her mother related to her father. She was controlling and assumed the dominant role in the marriage. He, on the other hand, passively accepted her control. She had always feared surrendering control and responsibility to a man, i.e., while flying, to the pilot. These earlier developmental factors contributed to the depth of her phobic anxiety.

Case 4. This was a male graduate student who was an accomplished athlete except for one activity. He had a morbid fear of swimming. When he was 11, he witnessed a drowning which so traumatized him that he could not bring himself to swim. Under hypnosis he was told that persons who swim well need not fear drowning. This patient knew swimming techniques. Under hypnosis he was told his body was like an inflated rubber raft, that his lungs, stomach, and bladder contained air so that when immersed, his body would easily float. He was also told that his arms and legs were like paddles. Further, he was told that at the first opportunity he would want to go to a pool and test out his "body raft." He did so immediately following the first treatment session and he realized to his amazement and pleasure that he could swim and float with no difficulty, and felt little anxiety. As he mastered the various swimming strokes and techniques, his anxiety disappeared and his phobia did not recur.

Case 5. This was a 33-year old married woman and mother of four who was obsessively preoccupied with death. It was revealed during hypnotherapy that she was deeply disturbed by the death of her mother whom she deeply loved. The patient was seven years old when her mother died. She remembered wanting very badly to visit her mother, a terminal cancer victim in the hospital, but she was not allowed to do so. Her mother was in great pain and relatives felt it would be too traumatic for the child to discover this. She wanted to attend the funeral, but this also was not permitted. To her then, her beloved mother was suddenly taken from her. She could not understand the meaning of death.

This patient was put into a deep hypnotic trance. She was then given suggestions that she did see her mother at the funeral. The patient wept as she envisioned the scene. It was further suggested that she would notice the beautiful serenity and peaceful expression on her mother's face. She was told that death for her mother meant a release from terrible suffering and that it was a real comfort to know that her mother didn't have to suffer any more. The funeral scene was recreated several times and each time the patient experienced less grief and anxiety and more composure and acceptance. She became more and more convinced that death meant a welcome relief from suffering. On her last visit and during hypnotherapy, the patient's expression was calm and serene. Death no longer occupied her thoughts and she became more cheerful and responsive to her husband and family.

These five cases are typical of the phobias which have been successfully treated by the use of hypnosis. Clinicians not too familiar with the hypnotherapy technique often question the depth and effectiveness of hypnosis for treating phobic and other states. They ask if there is a compensatory anxiety or habit formation arising from the psychic energy formerly invested in the phobia. In over five years' experience using hypnotherapy routinely in the treatment of phobic states, no such compensating anxiety has been manifested. Once the earlier causation or trauma has been discovered and thoroughly vented through hypnorevivification, and with attendant reassurance and suggestions of mastery and self-confidence, the phobia disappears with no recidivistic affect.

HYPNOSIS IN PSYCHIATRY: SPECIFIC CLINICAL INDICATIONS AND APPLICATIONS

Use of Hypnosis for Potentiations of Medication or Placebos

It should be stressed that the administration of drugs and placebos can often be made highly effective therapeutically when given in combination with hypnotic suggestion.

A 45-year old male came to the clinic complaining of nervous tension, anxiety, insomnia, anorexia and a general state of depressed affect. He had marked feelings of inadequacy, lacked drive and ambition and seemed rather despairing of the future. He told of how he had for several years become increasingly impotent and had considerable difficulty in maintaining an erection and that he had finally reached the point where he couldn't even attain an erection at all. He had been to two physicians to seek help. They had both prescribed Methyl Testosterone in considerable doses but this had not made it possible for him to overcome his problem. On occasion, the testosterone had given him an initial erection but he was unable to maintain it. In view of the doses of the hormone which he had received, it was clearly obvious that the patient like most such patients, was suffering from a functional disorder—psychic impotence. At this stage he was hypnotized and given placebo medication. He was then given suggestions that he would receive a medication which was imported from Peru and had been discovered accidentally by the natives there when they had observed that cattle eating a certain plant developed very strong sexual excitement and tended to breed a great deal. That this particular plant tended to not only cause strong and sustained erections but also tended to rapidly restore or activate the sexual functions to such an extent that an excellent state of virility was reestablished in a relatively short time; further that this herb extract not only markedly stimulated the sexual organs by means of causing a marked increase in blood flow but also in stimulating sex gland secretion and cellular proliferation, and acted as a releasing influence, thereby mobilizing a great deal of dammed up sexual feelings. The patient was carefully cautioned not to take an overdose of this powerful drug. It was suggested to the patient that the longer the medication acted on him, the better the result. To enhance suggestive influence, he was advised that there was often difficulty and time required in securing this rather rare and unusual preparation. Need I add that the results obtained were little short of miraculous in a number of such cases. Potency was rapidly restored in the majority of these cases of functional impotence. However, the greatest benefit noted was that the despair and depression disappeared as did the insomnia, anorexia, anxiety, and all the other symptoms. Above all, the patient was now convinced that he hadn't lost his manhood, but in fact, had, as in most cases, attained a potency which he had never had previously. Feelings of anxiety, inferiority and inadequacy were rapidly dissipated. Now that a very favorable rapport was established and the patient relieved of his unhappy preoccupation, objective efforts were made to pursue the underlying psychopathology of the condition. Certainly the great majority of these patients had been passive males, most of whom had marked castration anxieties and feeelings of anxiety about sexuality generally. All kinds of early traumas and parental mishandling of the rearing of their children, particularly with reference to sex behavior and development, was revealed. The placebo with which we had the highest success was E1. Iron, Quinine and Strychnine to which we would add a couple of drops of an herbal extract such as Gentiana. This hypnosis plus placebo technique has proved invaluable at our clinic in the successful treatment of large numbers of patients suffering from psychic impotence and frigidity.

However, the technique does not have to be limited to the administration of placebos alone. The actual pharmacological effect of many drugs, i.e., cortisone, various hormones, and particularly drugs which act upon the autonomic nervous system such as Bella Donna, Priscoline, ephedrine, caffeine, etc. may be potentiated by hypnotic suggestion.

Treatment of Frigidity

In general, one must differentiate between true frigidity and those conditions in which the female is reacting in a defensive manner because of frequent disappointment with and the inadequacy of her male partner. In the latter instance, the term "pseudo-frigidity" is often applied, referring to the failure of the male to perform and in general, due to a lack of knowledge concerning sexual relations. Generally these conditions can be alleviated by proper counseling and reeducation.

In true frigidity, one frequently encounters vaginismus, or painful and difficult intercourse. It is important to emphasize that often frigid women tend to project impotence on to their husbands. A typical case is that of a woman who had come in stating that her husband was sexually inadequate and unable to gratify her, and asking that he be given medication. Methyl testosterme linguets were given her husband. About ten days later, this patient called around 1:00 A.M. in a very disturbed state, exclaiming over the telephone, "For heaven's sake, Doctor, can't you get this man away from me? He's driving me crazy!" During a hypnotic trance, the woman admitted a long history of frigidity, and in considerable detail, described her early life; how her mother had been very disturbed about her marital relations with the father, how she had conveyed to the patient that she was being abused, and humiliated, and painfully so, and that a woman's life was one of miserable and unhappy submission. The patient came to dread the sexual experience, and to deeply resent the treatment of her mother by her father. Within herself a strong conviction grew that she would not ever permit any man to do this to her when she got married. Her deep-seated apprehension and revulsion toward coitus which was brought out fully under hypnosis, of course, explained why she had been so ambivalent and rejecting toward her husband on the one hand, and so deprecating and emasculating of him on the other.

The causes of frigidity vary considerably from more superficial causes to deep-seated neurotic conditions. In any case hypnoanalysis is a valuable tool in arriving at the basic etiology of the condition as well as in promptly aiding the patient. As was previously mentioned, very excellent results were obtained in the treatment of frigidity by the combination of direct suggestion and placebos, followed by hypnoanalysis and individual psychotherapy or group psychotherapy.

As Kroger so correctly stated with reference to the treatment of gynecological conditions of functional origin, it is very important to try to help the patient gain an awareness of her problems and to point out that in certain circumstances, she may have a recurrence of her condition, but that with patience and understanding, the condition will ultimately clear up entirely. The combined use of psychoanalytic methods and hypnosis may not only be an important time saver in the final resolution of many such deep-seated problems, but in many instances prove more effective. With hypnoanalytic technique, as pointed out, the improved transference relationship, the exploitation of hyperaffectivity, hyperamnesia, age regression, improved recollection of dreams, posthypnotic suggestion and even, when necessary, the induction of dreams and imagery by the use of post hypnotic suggestion which would center around specific conflicts, may contribute valuable insights into the basic causes of the illness and may aid patients to communicate their problems more freely and to follow through with the necessary treatment program.

As mentioned earlier, a valuable technique for uncovering repressed, painful feelings and experiences is "automatic writing" in which suggestions are given to the patient that they will spontaneously write about what is troubling them most or about certain traumatic experiences. Similarly, under hypnosis suggestions can be given to sketch the image they have of their parents, their employer, and significant persons in their life ("automatic drawing"). Interpretation of the writing and drawing should be obtained in both the hypnotic and waking states.

Treatment of Premenstrual Anxiety and Tension

This is often found correlated unconsciously with the fear of pregnancy. Aside from fear of missing the period is an aversion to and rejection of menstruation expressed in the term the "curse." Such attitudes are often found to be due to early faulty conditioning by a disturbed mother with unnatural, unhealthy attitudes toward sex, menstruation, femininity and motherhood. These patients often reveal unconscious fears of helplessness and of rejection. Many of these patients also reveal a kind of helpless, impotent rage at having been born into a female role and having to accept it even though they resented this role so strongly. Frequently premenstrual tension was associated with depression symptoms, and often followed by dysmenorhoea. Many patients, often during the menstrual or premenstrual period, may reveal such symptoms as gastrointestinal upsets, headache, urinary frequency, bladder pressure and general malaise, etc. One case in point was that of a 44-year old woman who revealed under hypnosis deep feelings of resentment, bitterness and frustration due to her husband's lack of consideration of her feelings and his neglect of her because of his involvements with business associates, club activities, which he felt were necessary for his business. As she had been reared under stern discipline, she found it very difficult to externalize her resentment and so turned these feelings inward. She thus developed a severe headache by means of which she sought to gain her husband's solicitude, understanding and compassion. In this instance, the hypnocathartic method was employed in which the patient was put into a medium deep trance and permitted to abreact her feelings in the presence of her husband. He was quite impressed with the sincerity of her outburst, and promised to cooperate in trying to relieve her distress. The tremendous insight gained by the husband in this instance was ultimately of immeasurable benefit, not only to the patient but to their children as well.

Treatment of Headaches

It is understandable that as a secondary result of headaches, and particularly migraine headaches, patients often develop marked apprehension concerning the onset of a severe headache, and that this constant fearful anticipation apparently plays an important role in reproducing the headache.

Headaches can usually be rapidly relieved by hypnotic suggestion. Patients can be taught self-hypnosis so that they can rapidly relieve pain and discomfort. Hypnotic and posthypnotic suggestion can be given to relieve acute migraine attacks but may also be employed to allay the dreaded anticipations of future attacks of migraine. The patient can be reassured that by being trained in self-relaxation and self-hypnosis so that he can prevent such attacks whenever he feels them coming on, the relief of this fearful apprehension is often enough to remove the attacks entirely.

A 58-year old male consulted me in regard to severe migraine attacks. He usually could ascertain when the attacks were coming on. He was trained in self-induction by the posthypnotic method. He succeeded in aborting the attacks before their acute onset. Interestingly, as he was usually able to prevent the onset of attacks, his apprehension of further attacks diminished markedly, and future attacks diminished greatly in frequency. It was clear that continual anxiety of another migraine attack kept him in a state of guarded apprehension.

Likewise, the positive anticipation of the patient that he can be helped over a longer period of time tends to reduce anxiety. This is highly important since excessive cumulative anxiety is often the cause of acute migrainous attacks. Of course, when headaches are fairly well localized, persistent and severe, the possibility of brain tumor needs to be ruled out–particularly, if other neurological signs are present, i.e., dizziness, unsteady gait, visual disturbances, sensory or motor disturbances, etc.

Positive anticipatory attitudes of patients greatly facilitate their response. This is well-illustrated by the fact, for instance, that patients often traveling long distances for therapy have arrived and almost spontaneously gone into a hypnotic trance. The anticipatory build-up was so tremendous in many instances that the therapeutic response was prompt.

Negative anticipatory influence must be avoided. For instance, if a resistive patient happens to be in the waiting room, and discourages the subject, resistance and negative anticipatory feelings and anxieties may develop. Stimulating, positive, motivational and anticipatory feelings in the patient can be most helpful. The interest of the patient should be aroused, if possible, particularly with reference to the benefits that they will observe in themselves as a result of the treatment, as well as pleasurable experience they will have. Having once enjoyed the tranquility and relaxation of the hypnotic trance, and awakening in a relaxed and pleasant state of mind, most patients eagerly look forward to being hypnotized again. It is in this connection wise not to emphasize to the patient that hypnosis is a cure-all or to make excessive claims. Further, it should not be encouraged as an escape from the reality situation. The therapist must always be on the alert not to permit the patient to become excessively dependent on him and the treatment. He must always point to the fact that the gains the patient will make and the real pleasures to be derived will be attained in the reality situation. This must be rigidly stressed; and that the hypnosis and post-hypnotic suggestion are merely for the purposes of helping the patient to enjoy reality to a greater extent and to fulfill his objectives in the real world in a satisfactory manner. In this connection, the potential capabilities and assets of the patient must be stressed, rather than to overemphasize the authority and strength of the therapist. The patient should be helped to develop a new concept of self incorporating self-acceptance, feelings of adequacy, pride in positive achievement, feelings of entitlement, as Camilla Anderson termed them. The patient needs to discover in himself his real capabilities, his authentic self, and a fuller degree of self-realization which will lead to greater achievement, success and happiness.

Treatment of Somnambulism

Once while I was working as a psychiatric consultant in a prison for adult males, a 27-year old prisoner who was disciplined and locked up for sleepwalking was referred to me. He was hypnotized and regressed to his first somnambulistic experience which occurred when he was 16. At the time he had a dream that the ghost of his highly authoritative, disciplinary grandfather was standing over his bed. He became terrified, arose, and began running until he was exhausted. Since then, at times, the ghost image has been obscured but the patient again feels the panic and runs.

Under hypnosis, he told of his fear of his grandfather, the fear of his punishment, i.e., locking him in the house for two to three days with no outside privileges. He also revealed how grandfather made him feel very guilty and unworthy. He was always fearful of punishment for if he got away from his grandfather, his mother would switch him. Under hypnosis he was made to confront his grandfather's ghost standing over him—to realize that he could not harm him and that he could tell his grandfather's image off. He did this to the point of venting his pent up resentment toward his grandfather fully. He was even able to laugh at and ridicule the grandfather's ghost. Since these past hurts and fears have been confronted and ventilated, the somnambulism has ceased. There is little doubt that the prison milieu—the feeling of being closed in-had been aggravating his condition.

Hypnosis in the Treatment of the Psychoses

The value of hypnosis in psychoses is limited. Where there is marked ego disorganization, the patient's concentration and attention may be difficult to maintain and induction may be difficult or impossible. In the treatment of psychotics, the primary aim is to increase rather than to decrease their awareness of reality. The psychotic usually has a fear of loss of direction and control. Since the hypnotic state involves a surrender of control, it can be detrimental. Obviously, the psychotic needs greater rather than lesser awareness and contact with reality. Hypnosis stimulates fantasies and suggestibility. The psychotic already is usually involved in excessive fantasies, which he generally regards as real because of his inability to discriminate between fact and fantasy, between reality and unreality. Heightened suggestibility tends to enhance paranoid delusions and ideas of reference.

In certain psychotic conditions in which the ego disorganization is less marked, such as in most depressive, manic-depressive, paranoid, or borderline schizophrenic states, hypnotic induction is often possible and may yield positive results. In the above cases, hypnosis may be particularly valuable in furthering communication and exploring deeply repressed conflicts. States of agitation and communication blocks can often be markedly relieved and recollection enhanced. The resultant emotional catharsis may be quite beneficial to the patient; however, the therapist must be careful not to consciously confront such patients with traumatic and conflict-laden revelations unless they are in such a state that they would be capable of handling these. Overloading the already damaged ego with additional emotional stress can precipitate serious psychotic reactions. In certain psychotic states, particularly schizophrenia, the patient is to varying degrees already quite dissociated and in trance-like hypnogogic states. Since in hypnosis and in psychosis, the unconscious tends to become conscious, fantasies and dreams may become realities to the patient. The division between conscious and unconscious is progressively lost and reality testing and discriminatory functions are reduced or absent. Hence, it is obvious that hypnosis is of little avail and could only further dissociative processes and lessen reality-testing capabilities. Moreover, dissociation interferes markedly with the concentration necessary for hypnotic relaxation.

In early schizophrenia, in instances where there is not yet too marked disintegration of the personality and where some degree of understanding and communication are still possible, hypnosis can be used to advantage. Here great care must be exercised, as aforementioned, not to overburden a patient with revelations and interpretations with which he cannot cope. Stress on the ego can be somewhat relieved by abreaction. Better insight into the etiology of the patient's illness can often be gained. The patient in many instances can be constructively motivated by means of posthypnotic suggestion into increased contact and communication with the outer world and in accepting treatment. Emotional blocks can be explored. Likewise, associations related to fantasies and symbol projections of the patient can often be elucidated. Hypnosis may be of value in furthering communications with withdrawn schizoid or borderline schizophrenic personalities who do not manifest overt hallucinations or delusions and with whom communication is almost always difficult. In applying hypnosis to such patients, it is important to use a sympathetic, warm and empathic approach to further rapport and cooperation when indicated. With paranoid patients a warm approach may arouse suspicion and it is better to be matter of fact and professional.

There are certain precautions that should be considered. In many instances, hypnosis yields best results, as aforementioned, by releasing pent-up tensions and inducing a pleasurable relaxed state. It is generally best not to probe traumatic conflicts too deeply and not to consciously ventilate disturbing material unless the therapist feels that the patient is prepared to handle it emotionally. Particularly with the schizophrenic it is wise to avoid the words "hypnosis" or "hypnotism" and to speak in terms of relaxation. As a matter of fact, this is done with most of our patients.

Hypnosis should be primarily used to calm, reassure and relieve anxieties and vent hostility, and not to stimulate fantasies. Patients can be influenced into greater social participation and, in some instances, hypnosis can be of considerable value in strengthening the transference relationship. If hypnosis is employed, it should be utilized with patients who are on medication and have a sufficient degree of reality contact and awareness.

Often under hypnosis it is possible to more readily determine the sources of mental stress in the environment of the patient so that these can be better dealt with. Sometimes it is possible to break up, alleviate or counteract delusions or psychotic fixations by use of strong hypnotic suggestion in which the patient is made to doubt or reject his psychotic fixations. The following case is illustrative.

A 70-year old female patient was suffering from a chronic paranoid condition, with persistent delusions over a period of years, that she was being subjected to bodily torture by means of psychic influences which she termed "psychic hypnosis." Since she was highly suggestible, it was possible to put her into deep trances and, by means of strong suggestion, to create artificial amnesia and blocks related to the persecutory symptoms. In place of these, pleasant, harmless preoccupations were substituted. It has been possible, as a result, to greatly relieve this patient's fear and suffering.

HYPNODRAMA

Hypnodrama can be a very useful technique, particularly when difficulties in communication are marked. Hypnotic relaxation, like psychodrama, markedly steps up affective response and memory. The emotional outpouring in hypnodrama is very intense and often quite revealing. Ego defenses and resistances are, for the most part, inactivated and overcome by the tremendous surge of feelings and protests experienced by the protagonist. Stimulation and provocation of the protagonist in the hypnodrama situation are experienced quite intensely, with corresponding strong reactions. Hypnodrama also tends to impress a psychodramatic audience because it is so deeply revealing and moving, and to the audience represents the true "deeper feelings of the person."

Due to the hyperaffectivity in the hypnotic state, I have found it very effective to create fantasy hypnodramas by suggestion so that the individual successfully confronts the dreaded situation, i.e., in altitude and flying phobias, in water phobias, attack violence phobias, claustrophobia, and many other specific fearful types of encounters. By repeatedly reliving the hypnodramatic experience in their fantasy without any emotional trauma, a progressive desensitization occurs which can rapidly resolve the phobic condition. When the resolution of conflicts and personality characteristics call for greater insight and recognition of repeated destructive patterns occurring, the results are best when posthypnotic psychodrama is used so that the protagonist can operate at the higher intellectual awareness and understanding level of consciousness. Posthypnotic suggestions are given that can greatly stimulate acting-out and catharsis.

The following case illustrates the value of hypnodrama as a therapeutic measure. This is the case of a 19-year old, white female, married and five months' pregnant, at the time separated from her husband. She was referred by a colleague who had had great difficulties in treating her, declaring that she was noncooperative, indifferent, and, in his opinion, an outright psychopathic personality. He felt she was unscrupulous and seriously lacking in conscience, and unable to develop any deep attachment towards anyone. He felt further resentful towards her, but was unaware, apparently, of his own resentment because she had seduced one of his other patients in a homosexual episode. Since she was quite uncommunicative, he asked me if I would hypnotize her. Previous attempts to hypnotize her by conventional methods had failed. She was relaxed without difficulty in less than five minutes by the endogenic method. She then revealed that she had lost her mother early, when about three, and that she then had a stepmother who, she felt, never loved her, and with whom she only recalled unhappiness. Her father, whom she loved dearly, was the only one in her life who, she felt, really cared for her; he died when she was seven. Her loving father appeared enshrined in her memory. She revealed that since her father's death, she had always been seeking the image of such a loving father in a man, but that she had never found him. She had begun to despair and to feel that there was no such person.

After a preliminary evaluation under hypnosis, it was decided, with the consent of her therapist, to have her act out her feelings in a hypnodrama. This was done on the same evening after the initial induction. She was given a posthypnotic suggestion that she act out her feelings about her marriage and her family after she awakened. Upon emerging from the trance, she readily entered into a psychodrama with the aid of auxiliary actors. In the hypnodrama she acted out the rejecting hostile stepmother in role reversal. She also acted out the events leading up to her ill-considered and unfortunate marriage and the motivations involved. In part, she was trying to escape from the painful situation with her stepmother and she was very unhappy and ashamed at not having an attractive home and many of the nice things she had always wanted. Her young prospective husband promised her everything. She pointed out that she could never have loved him because, after all, she loved the father she had enshrined, and there was no one like her father and there never could be. Tears at this time were evident. She further acted out her relationship to her therapist, adding that he could never be like her father. When asked why not, she stated, "Because he doesn't love me. I feel that he resents me, and that he treats me only because he feels sorry for me." She then went on in further discussion to point out that only a man who loved her could help her and that she would not act foolishly and destructively if she really felt loved by a kind father figure because she would want to please such a person by being the kind of person that he wanted her to be. The dramatic outpouring was quite impressive. The therapist came to understand his own countertransference feelings and why he had not succeeded in helping this patient after working with her for so long.

SUMMARY

In summation, therapeutic hypnosis can be an effective psychiatric technique in the following clinical areas:

1. Differential diagnosis (differentiating between organic and functional, i.e., hysteria, malingering conditions)
2. Therapy
   a. In promoting overall cooperation with treatment program
   b. In motivating the patient
   c. In aiding the patient in carrying out retraining/
   corrective exercises in cases of muscular weakness or limb impairment
   d. In encouraging patient to become mobile
   e. In instilling the will to get well

    f.   In improving rest and relieving discomfort and pain

3.   Exploring psychological factors (i.e., in clinging to symptoms for secondary gains; attention, sympathy; avoidance of responsibility, material and emotional dependency, escape from disagreeable persons, relationships, or situations; or because of fear of failure)

4.   In overcoming anxiety or fear in striving to overcome handicap

5.   In combating feelings of inferiority or rejection in the neurologically handicapped

6.   In retraining of the handicapped

Chapter 8

CLINICAL APPLICATIONS OF
HYPNOSIS IN VARIOUS SPECIALTIES

HYPNOSIS IN THE SPECIALTIES

The value of hypnosis in the specialties must be emphasized. Where clinical and operative procedures are particularly involved, there is always the element of apprehension and preoperative tension. Hypnosis can be effectively used to relieve such anxiety and tension, and is, of course, of particular value with children. The importance of hypnosis in relieving physical pain through hypnoanaesthesia and analgesia must be stressed. Often hypnosis can be effectively used for preparing the patient preoperatively, removing much psychic trauma and reducing shock, but also of making it possible to get better anaesthesia with less anaesthetic quantitatively. Hypnosis, because it has particular value in the immobilization of the patient, introducing not only sensory but motor inhibition, can be of great value in immobilizing the patient so that treatment may be carried

192

out more effectively and, in general, with less trauma to the patient (in cases where fractures require immobilization).

The use of hypnosis not only in relieving preoperative anxiety and tension and pain, but also for facilitating postoperative rest and reducing pain and discomfort is significant. Patients can be taught autohypnosis in those cases where it is necessary for them to relieve themselves repeatedly from attacks of discomfort, pain or insomnia, so that they can rest well and, thereby, make additional gains.

Hypnosis is becoming increasingly important in the various specialties, particularly in ophthalmology, as well as in ear, nose, and throat, urology, orthopedics, and other fields. An area of considerable importance for the application of hypnosis is that of removing phobias and resistances to treatment which may be based on earlier traumata. Furthermore, in general, the cooperation of the patient with the treatment regime and carrying out instructions can be greatly enhanced by hypnotic suggestion.

Hypnosis can be of great value in the various specialties in helping to differentiate hysterical and functionally etiological conditions from organic ones. Furthermore, it can be of considerable value in evaluating the nature of the emotional disturbances in patients and determining whether they require psychotherapeutic intervention. The overall value of hypnosis in reducing bleeding and also for its antiphlogistic effects which are becoming increasingly apparent should be noted.

Hypnosis is being used extensively in the practice of dentistry to relieve anxiety, to induce analgesia and relieve discomfort. It can be useful in dental repair, prosthetic work, fitting dentures as well as training patients to use them. It can be very useful in orthodontics, in relieving pain and discomfort, and in influencing the patient to carry out the instructions and cooperate in the treatment regime.

SOME USEFUL APPLICATIONS OF HYPNOSIS IN THE PRACTICE OF GENERAL MEDICINE

Hypnotic suggestion can be employed to reduce inflammatory reactions because of its antiphlogistic action. This effect appears largely due to vascular changes induced by psychic effects on the vasomotor innervation. There is definite clinical evidence that hypnotic suggestions can reduce inflammation and pain in peripheral neuritis, such as in cases of sciatica, herpes zoster, etc.

Hypnotic suggestion can effectively reduce anxiety and cardiovascular tension, slow pulse rate, lower blood pressure and induce mental relaxation. In cardiovascular conditions relaxation and sleep are most important. Since hypnosis is beneficial in relieving anxiety and tensions generally, it can be quite valuable in relaxing patients and inducing drugless sleep. Of greatest importance is the use of hypnosis to rapidly uncover the underlying sources of tension and anxiety. Since psychosomatic disorders are primarily due to blocked and unexpressed painful or disturbing feelings, the value of hypnocatharsis should not be underestimated.

Hypnosis, in the form of hypnoaversion therapy, can be used for the treatment of obesity and diet control generally in conditions such as diabetes, hypertension, cardiac disorders, gastrointestinal conditions, etc. Hypnoaversion treatment can also be used effectively in treating nicotinism and alcoholism.

As noted earlier, hypnotherapy can be of great value in the treatment of hypertension. It can be used not only to relax the patient but frequently to uncover sources of tension and in some instances to help in resolving these.

Hypnotherapy, generally, is of great value in the treatment of psychosomatic disorders, i.e., migraine, ulcer, bronchial asthma, mucous colitis, neurodermatoses, dysmenorrhea, etc. More recently, I have been able to reduce pain in rheumatoid arthritic patients. It appears that the effects of cortisone can be potentiated by means of hypnosis.

Hypnotic suggestion may be employed to encourage patients to carry out a prescribed treatment regime.

HYPNOSIS IN SURGERY AND ANAESTHESIOLOGY

Hypnosis can be an important aid in differentiating hysterical symptoms from those which are organic. Furthermore, it can be of value in recognizing and uncovering the causes of psychosomatic conditions such as peptic ulcer, mucous colitis, etc.

Hypnosis can be of great benefit in relieving preoperative anxiety and reducing preoperative shock and postoperative discomfort. It has been demonstrated that bleeding can be markedly reduced. If the anaesthetist wishes, hypnosis can be employed to greatly reduce the amount of anaesthesia required, particularly in suitable subjects who have been prepared by being hypnotized previously. As a matter of fact, some years ago I hypnotized a woman upon whom a Caesarian was done without the use of any anaesthesia. She felt no pain or discomfort whatsoever and the overall result was excellent.

It is now well-established that the psychic trauma prior to surgery is often of marked significance in the patient's ability to tolerate surgery. This is particularly in the sensitive patient predisposed to anxiety.

In emergency, military and accident surgery the factor of shock can often be preoperatively allayed by the skillful use of hypnosis.

Postoperative pain and discomfort can be relieved or ameliorated by hypnosis. In some instances, the patient can be instructed how to relieve himself by self-hypnosis.

Hypnosis can be of considerable value in various postoperative procedures such as removing sutures, changing dressings and removing drains, etc. Often hypnotic suggestion can be utilized at this time to allay subjective discomfort, pain, ventilate tensions and improve rest of the patient.

An important consideration is the application of hypnoanalgesia and anaesthesia in patients generally regarded as poor surgical risks, i.e., in cardiacs where respiration and circulation are impaired; in diabetic, uremic, tuberculous, hemophilic or patients with tendencies toward excessive bleeding. In the latter instance, the value of hypnosis in reducing bleeding can be exploited.

The possibility of postoperative complications such as bronchopneumonia, gaseous distension, nausea, emesis, hiccups which often complicate anaesthesia, can be in most instances eliminated when hypnoanalgesia and hypnoanaesthesia reduce or make unnecessary the use of anaesthetics. The occurrence of temporary or longer term paresis as a complication of spinal anaesthesia can also thus be avoided.

Another advantage of hypnoanaesthesia is that the patient can be instructed by the hypnotist to alter his respiration or position or to void as may be indicated.

Posthypnotic suggestion can be used effectively to influence the patient to carry out the doctor's instructions postoperatively, i.e., diet, medication, exercise, rest, etc. Hypnotic analgesia and anaesthcsia can be used in minor surgery either alone or in combination with topical anaesthetics, etc.

Hypnotized patients recover immediately. They are therefore able to partake of nourishment and medication earlier. The period of hospitalization may thus be shortened.

In 1958, I reported the use of a prolongation technique which has proved to be quite effective in prolonging hypnotic relaxation and preventing the patient from emerging from the trance.

The patient is instructed initially in the hypnotic trance that as long as he strives to remain in his hypnotized state, he will remain free of any discomfort whatsoever—and that he should not emerge from the trance until given specific instructions by his hypnotist or surgeon to do so and in that event he will then awaken feeling free of pain or discomfort.

Certainly not every patient is a ready subject for hypnosis, nor is hypnoanalgesia or anaesthesia indicated in all instances. However, a skillful hypnotist can readily hypnotize most patients without difficulty.

It must be kept in mind that not all patients can become hypnotically analgesic after the first induction. Frequently a second or third induction is required in order to deepen the hypnotic trance and obtain satisfactory analgesia. However, second and third inductions are relatively easy with proper technique and require but several minutes. Generally, it has been our experience that unless sufficient depth to obtain hand levitation is achieved, the analgesia will not be sufficient.

It is best to use strong suggestion to the effect that the patient will feel no pain. It is advisable to test the patient initially with a nonpainful stimulus. You can point out, "You see, you feel no pain whatsoever and your body is getting increasingly anaesthetic until soon you will feel absolutely nothing." Each time the patient is tested, the pressure of the pin or needle can be increased and the suggestion repeated, "You see—you are feeling less and less. Your anaesthesia is progressing beautifully. You can feel a slight pressure, but no pain—no pain."

Similarly, posthypnotic suggestion can be effectively utilized not only in deepening the trance but by adding, "The next time you enter into the hypnotic trance you will not only go much deeper but you will become increasingly more and more anaesthetic and feel no pain whatsoever."

Griffiths is quoted (by Ambrose and Newbold) to the effect that hypnosis is of value as an adjunct to anaesthesia because of the psychically calming effect of hypnosis, the induction of general anaesthesia may be smoother and that consequently, the amount of any chemical or physical anaesthetic is likely to be reduced. Further, hypnosis is of value, particularly in abdominal surgery where muscular relaxation is required.

Mention should be made of the observations of Goldie concerning the use of hypnosis in minor surgery in the casualty department of a hospital. Goldie sought to evaluate the use of hypnotic analgesia and anaesthesia with acute emergency cases both as an adjunct and as a substitute for conventional anaesthesia. He attempted to demonstrate a technique that is simple, practical and effective with untrained subjects. Goldie had little difficulty in inducing hypnosis and for instance reports that he treated 28 consecutive orthopedic cases in a single month and only failed to induce hypnosis sufficient for surgical reduction in two of them.

This certainly contrasts sharply with earlier reports that only 30 per cent of hypnotized subjects were capable of reaching anaesthesia. No worker in this field has achieved the successes reported by Goldie.

Bramwell, who was certainly a master of hypnotic technique concluded, "The chief objection to hypnotic anaesthesia is the difficulty and uncertainty of the induction of the necessary degree of hypnosis and generally hypnosis never becomes deep enough for operative purposes." He adds that, suggestive anaesthesia can only be induced in about ten per cent of those hypnotized.

Ambrose and Newbold have made it a practice to give patients achieving medium or deep hypnosis cards which they can present to their doctors or dental surgeons—should they require hypnosis for minor surgery, etc. They have found it feasible with many of their patients to use posthypnotic suggestion that they would upon request of the doctor or dentist (and nobody else) suggest to themselves the counting of numbers of up to five or ten—on reaching this number they could achieve a light hypnotic trance. This trance could then be deepened by the doctor pressing gently with his index finger on the patient's forehead. The patient is trained to awaken by counting forward to five slowly. We have the patient count backwards as he goes under and forward as he merges from trance. Thus, doctors or dentists can be put in rapport with their patients.

The studies of Finer on repose to ischemic pain was able to demonstrate an increased tolerance to pain while subjects were under the influence of posthypnotic suggestion.

The value of hypnotic anaesthesia and analgesia for minor surgical and dental procedures in children should be stressed. For instance—Ambrose and Newbold point to the ease with which deep hypnosis can be readily achieved in children, stating that over 60 per cent can obtain deep hypnosis and thus analgesia for simpler surgical procedures such as lumbal puncture—venesections—incisions, etc. Of particular value is the use of hypnotic relaxation in children preoperatively, i.e., in tonsillectomies, appendectomies, etc. following which inhalation anaesthetics can be employed. In such instances less drug or gas anaesthetic is required to attain satisfactory analgesia.

Ambrose and Newbold also point to the high percentage of patients who can attain a deep state of hypnosis on the very first induction. They claim that one in four can accomplish this in favorable circumstances. Such results, in the author's opinion, could only be attained by a skilled and experienced hypnotist. It is perhaps more to be regarded as a goal to shoot at by those new in the art.

In summary, hypnosis in surgery offers the clinician invaluable adjunctive assistance, especially in the following treatment áreas:

a. In relieving preoperative anxiety
b. In reducing bleeding
c. In relieving pain and nausea postoperatively
d. In furthering rehabilitative measures and increasing cooperation of patient, especially in disabilities and in orthopedic cases
e. In relieving or reducing pain in minor surgical procedures
f. In differential diagnosis

Hypnosis in Obstetrics

Since hypnosis has proven to be of significant importance in obstetrics, I have taken the liberty of dealing with that subject at some length. Furthermore, in view of the fact that hypnotherapy is of such value in treating gynecological problems, I have also devoted more attention to that subject. Frequently, the emotional factors underlying certain gynecological conditions can be rapidly elicited while the individual is in a hypnotic trance. Often refractory conditions such as frigidity, vaginismus and dysmenorrhea can be rapidly resolved.

One of the first to recognize the great value of hypnosis in obstetrics was the late eminent obstetrician J. B. DeLee. Among others who made significant contributions in this area were Kroger, Freed, Read, Abramson, Heron, Schneck, Newbold, and others.

The primary clinical advantages appear to be the following: greater muscular relaxation, improved labor, shortening of delivery time, relief of pain and discomfort, without use of drugs or anaesthetics, and better placental separation, reduced postpartal bleeding, and the marked reduction of stillbirths. Important is the fact that under hypnosis the mother can experience childbirth as a joyful fulfilling nontraumatic experience.

The application of hypnosis to obstetrics can be divided into three phases: The prenatal period, the labor period, and the postpartum period.

I shall first discuss the advantages to be gained in the prenatal period. By means of hypnosis and hypnotic suggestion, it is not only possible to relieve many symptoms of discomfort during pregnancy but also to facilitate the cooperation of the obstetrical patient in carrying out the prescribed regimen of the obstetrician, with reference to such matters as proper exercises, diet, avoiding excessive strain or trauma, getting proper rest, and cooperating with the doctor in faithfully adhering to his instructions regarding regular medical check-ups and medication.

In many instances, patients who are unfamiliar with the use of obstetrical hypnosis may have some apprehension and resistance to its use. I have found that the simplest expedient for overcoming this is to tell the patient that I would like to evaluate her capacity for muscular relaxation. She is then given muscular relaxation exercises and tests by means of the endogenic method and usually relaxed initially without difficulty into a hypnotic trance. Following the initial induction, anxiety is dissipated and patients are generally both willing and cooperative with the procedure. With each successive induction, the patient is able to relax more deeply and attain a greater degree of analgesia and anaesthesia. I have found that many patients can be trained in autohypnosis, which of course, has the added advantage that the patient can practice deepening the trance at home and that, should the obstetrician be absent or delayed at the onset of labor, the patient can readily relax herself and experience no discomfort whatsoever. Many patients have attained such a high degree of ability to relax themselves to an analgesic level that they can accomplish this within one to three minutes. This method has in our experience and in that of other investigators, such as Schneck, Kroger, and Newbold, proven to be clinical practical and effective in many cases.

Use of Autohypnosis and Posthypnotic Suggestion

The endogenic technique of autohypnosis in my opinion is the most practical. The autorelaxation should be maintained until the completion of labor. Helpful in this regard is my prolongation technique (described in Chapter four). Autohypnosis is carried out as in the following example of a 24-year old primagravida who was referred by her obstetrician. The patient was four months pregnant at the time. The advantages of hypnosis in childbirth were discussed during the first session. The patient rapidly developed rapport and was quite cooperative. During the latter part of the first session, she was told that a practice hypnotic relaxation would be attempted. She was then promptly relaxed by the endogenic method. It was possible during the first session to deepen the trance by reverse counting and hand levitation. The patient was then seen a week later and again hypnotized. In the hypnotic trance, she was given the precise instructions of her obstetrician for cooperation during the prenatal period. The patient was then given posthypnotic suggestion to the effect that she would carry out autohypnotic relaxation exercises precisely according to instructions and was taught to awaken herself from the trance by means of counting from one to 20—she would awaken at the 20th count. Thus she would induce and deepen her trance by reverse counting and bring herself out of it by forward counting. The patient was able to rapidly induce self-hypnosis with a marked degree of hypnoanalgesia and anaesthesia during her first self-induced trance. She was given pain tests by her obstetrician and experienced no pain whatsoever. This patient has continued to practice self-induction two to three times weekly with the object of increasing the rapidity and depth of hypnosis as well as for purposes of relaxation. She was also instructed in the prolongation technique during her initial trance. This patient was told that following the onset of labor, she would maintain herself in the hypnotic trance and would not emerge until so instructed by her doctor or nurse. As long as she remained in the trance, she would experience no pain or discomfort whatsoever, but if she permitted herself to emerge, she would have to endure the pain which she was trying to avoid. This prolongation procedure has been employed by me successfully not only in prolonged labor but in major surgery, including a Caesarean operation performed at our hospital at Howard University by Drs. Thompson and Bradford under my directions in 1956.

The following case is an example of the application of hypnosis to obstetrics. The first session was had with the patient when she was five months pregnant. She was hypnotized by the endogenic method. During this session, she was given posthypnotic suggestion with reference to her diet, cooperation with her obstetrician's regime, and necessary exercises which he had recommended, etc. During the second session, the trance depth was increased by backward counting and hand-levitation. She had complained of some pressure on the bladder and lower spine and rectal region. Suggestions were given in which she was told that the pressure would soon disappear and the rationale given that the pelvic area and abdomen were accommodating themselves to the fetus and the enlarging uterus. This subjective feeling of pressure soon cleared up. She was seen twice monthly and with each visit it was easier to induce hypnosis. After the third visit, she relaxed deeply within two minutes, and was completely analgesic. Her labor be-

gan at 11 P.M. at approximately term. There was no difficulty in inducing a trance, a deep trance being attained in
less than two minutes. During the course of labor, she
cooperated fully, bearing down as she was given hypnotic
suggestions. She relaxed beautifully between pains; there
was no apprehension or any visible discomfort. She delivered at 2:30 A.M.; there was no evidence of any discomfort,
and the infant respired immediately after delivery. She
dilated beautifully, and no episiotomy was necessary. She
was told that she would be able to witness the birth of her
baby as she desired and to hear its first cry and that she
would remain free of pain. She expressed great joy at the
opportunity to see her baby being born and to be aware
that the baby had begun breathing promptly after birth.
During the progress of labor, she was able to feed herself,
to urinate, to carry on conversations with her husband and
the nurse, as well as with her attending obstetrician. Her
recovery following delivery was very prompt and uneventful. Placental separation was excellent, with little postpartum bleeding evident. This patient stated that at no time
had she felt any pain or discomfort whatsoever and was in
an excellent mood.

BENEFICIAL EFFECTS OF BREAST FEEDING

As was indicated earlier, the secretion or flow of breast milk
is very much affected by psychogenic factors. We feel, as
pointed out earlier, that the intimate contact between
mother and infant during the very early postpartum period,
as well as later, is of very great importance. This is under-
lined by Benedek who described the continued symbiosis
during the postpartum period between mother and infant
and feels that it affects the hormonal process. Mohr reports
that a patient had reported sudden inability to nurse following emotional excitation. While under hypnosis, she

was given suggestions that on the way home she would feel milk flow from her breasts. Within an hour she was having normal milk flow and had no recurrence of her difficulties.

Liebeault and Bernheim have reported many instances in which the flow of milk could be stopped or increased through hypnosis. This has also been supported by other investigators such as Goll, Heyer, and others.

PRENATAL

During the prenatal period, hypnotic and posthypnotic influence can be used further to encourage proper diet and exercises, care of teeth, avoidance of excessive physical and mental strain, taking necessary medications, for the relief of nausea and vomiting, and to encourage and prepare the mother to breast feed her child.

DURING LABOR

During the period of labor, hypnotic relaxation can be helpful in furthering pelvic and vaginal muscle relaxation. Better dilation and uterine contractions can be obtained largely because of the avoidance of sedation and analgesia. Furthermore, uterine as well as abdominal muscle contractility can be accentuated by hypnotic suggestion. Complete relief of anxiety, subjective discomfort and pain can be readily attained. All in all, there is far less stress on the patient due to these aforementioned factors of better pelvic muscular relaxation and dialtion, and the improved uterine and abdominal muscle contractions, thus shortening the labor period and facilitating delivery. The excellent relaxation of the patient and the avoidance of toxic drugs and anaesthetic can be of considerable value in delivering patients suffering from toxemia of pregnancy, cardiovascular disorders, or excessive anxiety. In this connection, I should like to mention the following case of a 40-year old woman, whom I encountered in the university obstetrical clinic while on a visit in Padua, Italy, who was suffering from a marked cardiac insufficiency. She was already somewhat decompensated and her obstetricians felt that it might be hazardous to give her sedation or anaesthesia. The marked tension and anxiety of the patient presented a problem. I hypnotized the patient without difficulty, the instructions being given through an interpreter who relayed them to the patient in Italian. This patient was able to have her baby a day later under hypnoanalgesia, without complications, and experienced no subjective discomfort.

SIMULATION AND ACTING-OUT UNDER HYPNOSIS

The following is a case of a 20-year old female who had expressed the desire to have her child under hypnosis.

For a number of sessions this patient permitted herself to enter only a light hypnotic trance. Analgesia could not be achieved. In investigating the causes of her defense reaction, she stated the following: "I am afraid to fully give up conscious control and an awareness of others around me." When an explanation of this reaction was further pursued, the patient stated that all through her childhood her mother had repeatedly told her of what a bad time she had had in labor and that she "should not have trusted those doctors." Her mother had thus created an obsessive fear within her surrendering control of her faculties and submitting to the instructions of a doctor. Her apprehension was understandable. Out of sheer anxiety, she even attempted to simulate a deeper hypnotic trance. However, it was obvious that she had not attained a deep enough state since she had failed to achieve analgesia. A conscious discussion of her underlying anxieties and their causes plus a reassuring sympathetic attitude on the part of the therapist made it possible soon after several sessions to put her into a deep hypnotic trance and to attain the desired analgesia.

It is interesting to note to what extent patients are capable of acting out in lighter states of hypnosis. There are some authorities who believe that hypnosis itself is an acting out phenomenon and in a sense the subject can enter into the hypnodrama as deeply as the subject desires. This patient was taught autohypnosis by means of posthypnotic suggestion. This was done in case the hypnotist was not available at the time labor began.

Of interest was the fact that the obstetrician who performed the delivery called me afterwards. He was quite amazed since he had had to apply high forceps because the umbilical cord was strangling the child. As a result of the rapid forceful delivery, the patient suffered an extensive perineal tear requiring considerable suturing. The obstetrician informed me that the patient awakened afterwards precisely as I had instructed her only when told that the operation was finished and she could come out of the trance. She had awakened smiling and relaxed, and immediately asked to see her baby. She stated that she had been completely free of pain or discomfort even though she had received no hypnotics or anaesthetics whatsoever.

POSTPARTUM EFFECTS

As a result of improved uterine and abdominal contractions, good placental separation is usually achieved, thus greatly reducing the possibility of the postpartum hemorrhage or infection. Bleeding, generally, is markedly reduced. Significant, also, is the improved subjective well-being of the patient and the overall faster recovery, reducing the period of hospitalization. Further, during the postpartum period, hypnosis can be used effectively to facilitate the milk flow.

BENEFICIAL EFFECT TO CHILD

The most significant advantage for the new-born child in the use of hypnoanalgesia to facilitate delivery is the fact that respiration is usually prompt and vigorous, due to the absence of respiratory depressant drugs and anaesthestics. Thus, a marked reduction in the incidence of still births can be achieved. It is now well established that prompt respiration and adequate oxygen supply to the new-born child is highly important in preventing often irreversible brain damage. Barcroft has demonstrated that even a mild, transient anoxia could cause cellular damage in the central nervous system, since brain cells are highly susceptible to damage from oxygen deficiency, more so than any other tissue in the body. Convulsions have been produced experimentally in pups whose mothers had received an insufficient amount of oxygen during labor. The extent to which such a deficiency might play an important etiological role in such conditions as idiopathic epilepsy, mental deficiency, aphasia, sensory as well as motor impairment, has been established. It is clear that due to the improved muscular relaxation and dilation, there is a lessening of the possibility of fetal injury. Passage of the fetal head is thus facilitated, lessening the possibility of brain injury. In instances where there is a breech presentation under hypnosis, there is less possibility of injury such as fracture or dislocation of the limbs. With the facilitation of labor and improved muscular relaxation, forceps deliveries should become less frequent, and in those instances where necessary, may be made easier.

Further clinical observation will answer the question as to whether the use of hypnosis in obstetrics may also reduce the incidence of Caesarian Section. One of the notable advantages that obstetricians have found with the use of hypnoanalgesia is that when necessary a small, painless episiotomy can be made to ease and speed up delivery. Ambrose and Newbold have wisely pointed to the value of hypnosis and its application to the delivery of premature babies. They correctly point to the fact that in such cases the risk of damage from asphyxia and trauma is greater than in those babies who go to term. They also point to the great need of premature babies for human breast milk. Certainly it is usually considerably more difficult to initiate respiration in a premature new-born. The absence of drugs and anaesthetics in such instances may be decisive.

Not to be forgotten is the gratification, in many instances, which the mother experiences from her awareness of the birth of the child. Hypnoanalgesia makes it possible for the mother to escape the pain and discomfort, but to enjoy the pleasures of childbirth. Hypnotic suggestion can be employed to both encourage the mother to breastfeed the baby, and to psychologically stimulate a more abundant flow, thus contributing greatly not only to the general health and development of the new-born child, but also to the mental well-being and emotional gratification of the mother. Breast-fed babies not only reveal a higher degree of resistance and immunity to infections and illnesses but also rarely suffer from disturbances of the gastrointestinal tract or skin conditions. One cannot ignore here the factor that the physical closeness of the mother to the child, and the gratification of the instinctual need of the infant to suckle at the mother's breast, is of considerable importance in the emotional development of the child. Similarly, breast feeding can be significant to the emotional well-being and physical health of the mother. The natural flow and disgorgement of the breast tends to reduce inflammatory and cystic breast conditions. Furthermore, many mothers develop anxiety and guilt feelings about their not breast feeding, or being separated from their infant.

In general, most obstetrical patients can be readily

hypnotized by well-trained practitioners in this art. (Contraindications with regard to the use of hypnosis are discussed in Chapter 10.)

Hypnosis can be quite helpful in the treatment and relief of a number of conditions occurring in pregnancy. Particularly valuable in this regard is the application of hypnotherapy to disorders involving the gastrointestinal tract, such as nausea, vomiting, hyperacidity, and flatulence. Organs enervated by the autonomic nervous system are readily influenced by hypnotic suggestion. The following case is illustrative: A 39-year old patient who was in her fourth month of pregnancy was having severe emesis, so severe that she had to be hospitalized. The diagnosis established was pernicious vomiting of pregnancy. The vomiting was promptly controlled by means of hypnotic relaxation and the exploration into the cause of her condition was attempted. She revealed that she was acutely disturbed over her husband's apparent coldness and indifference to her. Of late he had been quite preoccupied with other matters, and had neglected her, although he did find the time to devote himself to the interests of their 15-year old daughter. She began to feel increasingly insecure in her relationship with him as her pregnancy advanced. As the disturbance within her mounted, she began to have doubts about wanting to bear the child. Her husband was unable to understand what was occurring and offered neither reassurance nor support. Finally, she began to feel a strong desire to expel the child, which she repressed from consciousness, since she was not consciously aware of this impulse. While in a deep trance she gave expression to her impulse to reject and vomit out the fetus and the underlying reasons, the emotional disturbances giving rise to this impulse. His rejection of her caused her to feel a desire to reject the unborn child. She was given a strong posthypnotic suggestion that she would no longer feel the desire to vomit and that she would freely discuss the whole problem with the doctor following her awakening from the trance. The conflicts were then consciously ventilated, with her gaining insight and relieving a great deal of pent-up tension. A consultation was held with the husband who was then able to gain insight into her needs, and who as a result became more attentive and understanding in his attitude. The patient had an uneventful pregnancy thereafter with no further recurrence of vomiting.

Disturbing symptoms such as hyperacidity and flatulence frequently are of psychogenic origin and can often be greatly relieved by an exploration during the hypnotic trance of the underlying tensions as well as by direct suggestion. Patients frequently complain of lower abdominal pressure and urinary frequency. Such pressure symptoms often include complaints of backache which generally increase as term approaches. Considerable relief can be achieved when anxiety is a markedly contributing factor to the above conditions. Patients may be disturbed by fears of premature labor or threatened abortion. As indicated earlier, psychological as well as physical trauma may induce miscarriage or abortion. In such cases, prolonged hypnotic relaxation may be of value. Hypnosis can also be used to relieve the mental tension by means of catharsis.

In instances in which patients attempt to artifically abort, hypnosis can be employed to better evaluate the underlying emotional conflicts and the mental health of the patient.

Patients suffering from obesity and compulsive eating can often be helped by means of hypnotherapy, as for example, in the following case of a 30-year old primigravida who was in her fifth month of pregnancy. (See section on hypnoaversion therapy, Chapter 9). Her physician had referred her because she had been eating uncontrollably, was up to about two hundred pounds and showed increased blood pressure. He feared that her overweight condition might make her labor more difficult. This patient was in the habit of eating snacks between meals and of amassing considerable amounts of food to eat prior to retiring at night. Under hypnosis, it was found that she was suffering from a great deal of tension primarily centered around the fact that her husband showed little affection and attention at a time when she felt that she needed his emotional support most. She stated that she felt comforted when she ate and that it was a kind of oral pacifier, very much like putting the nipple in the mouth of a disturbed infant to relax him. She characterized her husband as a rather nondemonstrative person who showed little external feeling. The problem was attacked, not only from the point of view of attempting to help her husband gain insight into her emotional needs, but also by means of creating a hypnotically conditioned aversion to the high caloric foods that she craved most. This was achieved in several sessions and periodically reinforced. The approach proved to be quite successful, and as the patient was able to gradually reduce, her hypertension diminished. While dieting, she was given posthypnotic suggestion to the effect that she would supplement necessary vitamins and minerals to her diet which she did faithfully.

Pruritis sometimes occurs in pregnancy, a condition which may be caused by toxic factors, at times physical, such as stretching of the abdominal skin in advanced pregnancy. Psychological factors may also cause such itching and skin irritations. Itching and "crawling" may occur as a result of circulatory disturbances, particularly in the regions of the abdomen and lower extremities. The condition, if psychogenic in origin, generally responds promptly to suggestive therapy. It is important to explore the emotional basis of any tension, the contributing, underlying problems involved, and consciously ventilate these. In the meantime, symptomatic relief of symptoms can often be effectively relieved by a combination of medication or placebos plus hypnotic suggestion.

INSOMNIA

One of the most frequent disturbing problems in pregnancy is that of sleeplessness, since proper rest is an important part of the prenatal regime. The most common cause of insomnia in these cases is anxiety. This is manifested primarily by difficulty in falling asleep. I have found that fears of death of mother or child may prevail. In some instances, insomnia is associated here with the subconscious fear of abandonment, loss of love, etc., particularly when the husband is not too attentive or solicitious during the prenatal period. In some cases insomnia is attributable to such factors as urinary frequency, fetal movements, backache, etc. I have found that training the patient in autohypnosis has been often quite effective in relieving this problem. With those patients who tend to awaken during the night, my relaxation prolongation technique has been quite helpful.

In cases where there is malposition of the fetus, hypnoanalgesia may be quite helpful in performing an external cephalic version. Version is facilitated because of the greater degree of general relaxation and particularly the muscular relaxation of the patient. Hypnotherapy can be of benefit in calming patients suffering from hypertension, thyrotoxicosis, paroxysmal tachychardia, and other conditions. Often emotional disturbances which are found associated with these conditions can be resolved and the condition of the patient markedly improved.

HYPNOANAESTHESIA AND ANALGESIA

It should be emphasized that although hypnosis had been attempted many years ago in obstetrics procedures, the advent of inhalation anaesthesia and analgesia played an important part in discouraging the further application and clinical study of hypnosis in obstetrics. This is understandable when we consider some of the principal objections which were so well outlined by Owen Flood. Obstetricians have sought a simpler, more effective and reliable way to treat the average patient. As Owen Flood pointed out, the individual's susceptibility to hypnosis varied, it was time consuming, and at that time, of course, techniques for hypnotic induction and for maintaining hypnosis were not as well developed. Furthermore, the marked physiological and clinical advantages of hypnoanalgesia and anaesthesia were also not fully understood. It is regrettable that at that time, investigators did not pursue the real advantages that could have been gained by combining hypnoanalgesia and anaesthesia with inhalation anaesthesia as was referred to in the previous section on the subject. Mention at this point should be made of the work of Kroger and DeLee who are to be credited for their excellent insight into the possibilities of hypnosis in obstetrics. Kroger had observed quite correctly that following the use of deleterious drugs for inducing anaesthesia and analgesia in obstetrical patients, the fetus may suffer from anoxia. He points out further that it is well known that even a normal labor without anaesthesia or analgesia may be complicated by asphyxia. Certainly, it is well established that anaesthetic drugs may effect the fetus due to transfer through the placental circulation. We have already discussed the effects of these drugs on fetal respiration and circulation, showing how they can significantly increase the possibility of still birth. It is sometimes difficult for obstetricians and anaesthesiologists to avoid excessive drugging of the patient since the dosage requirements and the tolerance for various drugs and anaesthetics for individual patients may vary considerably.

Further, it should be emphasized that once the patient receives barbituates, sedative drugs, or anaesthesia, the patient's condition can no longer be as effectively controlled by the physician. However, if the patient is under hypnosis, it is possible to favorably influence respiration and muscular relaxation. Through the use of hypnosis in obstetrics, uterine contractions can be improved and the cooperation of the patient, in general, can be gained in a way that facilitates, shortens, eases labor. Both Owen Flood and Kroger have provided an excellent critique of the primary advantages and disadvantages of the use of hypnosis in labor.

Hypnoanaesthesia and analgesia provide a safe method, and the combined use of hypnosis and inhalation anaesthesia in the opinion of the author is the method of choice. Reference at this point is made to the excellent observations of Marmor who had very extensive experience in hypnoanaesthesia and who has recommended the giving of ether, for example, or a suitable inhalation anaesthetic, at the time when crowning or presentation of the fetus occurs. He pointed to the advantages, namely, that better relaxation could be obtained during the very important phase of delivery, that there was very little likelihood of the patient emerging from the trance which had occasionally occurred at this point in labor, and that if an episiotomy or other intervention were necessary to expedite delivery, this can be easily done and the necessary repairs quickly effected. We again stress this approach because as mentioned earlier, the administration, for example, of ether, in small amounts does not depress fetal or maternal respiration, but may even improve it. Furthermore, small amounts of anaesthetics do not cause any serious postpartal discomfort. Certainly, hypnosis reduces all danger as far as respiratory failure is concerned. Hypnosis offers the possibility of achieving painless natural childbirth.

In obstetrical hypnoanalgesia, there are such factors to consider as the degree of affective excitement of the mother during childbirth. There are occasions when the mother instinctively and emotionally strongly desires to experience the birth of her child and may even make strenuous efforts to awaken from the trance. She can be given suggestions to open her eyes and see her baby being born and experience the joyous thrill of having her baby. In such instances, I have found it best to give posthypnotic suggestions, that should the patient awaken from the trance spontaneously, she will feel no pain or discomfort—a technique recommended by Erickson. Marmor recommended a little anaesthesia be given at the moment of presentation of the head, crowning and delivery, particularly if an episiotomy is intended. Marmor's suggestion has proven to be clinically practical as a routine procedure.

Autohypnosis in obstetrics should be used selectively with suitable patients for several reasons. That it requires a longer period of prenatal training of the patient is not of major consideration. It is in my opinion contraindicated in patients suffering from deeper emotional disturbances; it could lead to pathological escapism and further dissociative tendencies.

It is far more advisable for the obstetrician or the anaesthetist utilizing hypnosis to be present and observe, and if necessary, control the state of the patient. This reduces anxiety. The hypnotic transference and rapport are important to the feelings of security and relaxation of the patient. The hypnotherapist can deepen the trance whenever necessary and sort of "play it by ear."

Autohypnosis can be used in a modified form in many cases. That is, after an initial induction by the hypnotist, the patient has been taught to deepen and maintain her relaxation by means of autosuggestion. Autohypnosis, as previously indicated, can be very effectively used with certain patients. Again, it is advisable to give a little anaesthesia during the period of crowning and delivery. Smaller amounts of ether, like alcohol, generally stimulate rather than depress respiration.

Autohypnosis can be employed in two ways: (1) By training the patient to carry out a modified endogenic routine. This procedure is effective with certain highly suggestible patients. For details see section on self-induction; (2) By posthypnotic suggestion and instruction. I prefer the latter as it is simpler and more rapid.

The following is an excellent case report by Schneck illustrating the use of autohypnosis:

A primigravida, aged 22 years, was first seen when about two months pregnant. At this visit the question of hypnosis during labor was discussed with her and her husband, since both had expressed a wish that this method of analgesia should be used for the confinement. It was explained that the essentials of the method were (1) to aim at the greatest possible degree of mental and physical relaxation so that labor became much easier and delivery was facilitated, and (2) to help her gain increased control over the functioning of her own body by establishing a positive and healthy attitude of mind towards the subject. The mechanism of labor was also explained to her in simplified terms.

After the ground had been thus prepared a simple suggestibility test was performed—although this is by no means essential—so that some idea could be obtained of the patient's possible response to hypnosis. Since this proved satisfactory she was seated comfortably in an armchair and told to commence regular breathing; at the same time suggestions of increasing relaxation were given as previously described. After ten minutes or so it was noticed that she was appreciably more relaxed and seemed rather drowsy. She was then given suggestions that as she continued to breathe quietly the relaxation would increase and that she would be able to relax in a similar manner during the birth of her baby. It was also suggested that she would keep perfectly fit and well throughout the whole of her pregnancy. At the end of half an hour the session was terminated by telling her to awaken slowly when she heard the number three being counted; this was followed by an assurance that she would feel perfectly normal and that any feeling of drowsiness or lethargy would rapidly disappear.

The patient was then seen at approximately monthly intervals until the sixth month, and then forthnightly during the seventh and eight months. There was a definite increase in the depth of relaxation with growing practice and, by the time the fourth session was reached, good analgesia to pin-prick was also obtained. This patient was not a somnambulist and always remembered all, or most, of what was said to her during the hypnotic state. By the sixth interview she was able to induce a moderate depth of hypnosis herself by following the same technique.

During the course of this prenatal training the following suggestions were given to her frequently:

1. That she would continue to keep fit and well
2. That everything was perfectly normal (as indeed it was)
3. That she would experience the contractions of her womb during labor as reasonably pleasant sensations
4. That she would be able to bring about great muscular relaxation herself, so that womb and the birth passages dilated to the fullest extent and thus made plenty of room for the baby to pass through easily
5. That she would be able to breast feed her baby satisfactorily as a good supply of milk would be available for this purpose

This particular patient was booked for hospital confinement, since she was a primigravida, and it was impressed upon her not to delay unduly in going to the hospital once she had reasonable grounds for believing she was in labor. She was also given the suggestion that she would have some initial discomfort from the early contractions so that she would have sufficient warning of the onset of labor; as soon as their significance was appreciated, and it was safe to do so, she would be able to induce a satisfactory condition of hypnosis and from then onwards experience the contractions as pleasant. The medical hypnotist who undertakes the training of obstetric patients must always take "Safety" as his watchword, and exercise extreme care in the framing of his suggestions.

Twelve days after the estimated date of delivery the patient went into labor and the results of her antenatal preparation was most gratifying. She suffered no distress during the first stage and, had she not been specially warned, might easily have not realized that she was in labor. During this period, when contractions were occurring every three minutes or so, the discomfort was so slight that she later stated, "I felt quite unconcerned, and almost wondered if the baby really was on the way." Throughout the second stage she relaxed extremely well and cooperated fully and without difficulty with the midwife who was responsible for the delivery. The only time she experienced any definite pain was at the moment of the crowning and delivery of the head, when the vulval outlet was stretched to its greatest extent. The baby, which weighed seven lbs. 11 ozs., was delivered in a good condition and the third stage was perfectly normal. In all, labor lasted between nine and ten hours and at no time were drugs of any kind administered. The puerperium was uneventful and the baby on discharge was purely breast fed. Later, the patient declared that she felt perfectly fit the moment the baby was born and expressed herself as most satisfied with her experience.

HYPNOSIS IN GYNECOLOGY

Dynamic psychiatry today was given ample evidence of sexual problems in the etiology of gynecological conditions. It is understandable that such functional conditions are often referrable to the sexual areas, particularly the pelvic area, in the female. Certainly these conflicts are not usually of recent origin, but go back into the life history of the patient, the type of rearing and emotional conditioning, particularly with respect to instruction or lack of instruction in matters of procreation, menstruation, motherhood, the role of a wife, and in general, acceptance of the female role. Roles are learned from the teaching and behavioral models that parents present to children. Parents who make one another unhappy and vent their frustrations, bitterness and rage on each in interminable repetitive conflicts obviously present destructive and discouraging models for their children. How can one build a good house with a faulty blueprint? Often parents who lack love for each other and feel trapped in the responsibilities of a marriage and children often turn to their children for the emotional support and companionship they need. Frequently, the father turns toward the daughter, the mother toward the son and this usually sets the stage for the "electra" and "oedipal" complexes.

Disturbances and traumatic situations that occur, particularly during puberty and adolescence often play an important role in the etiology of certain gynecological conditions. As indicated earlier, not only can the patient be helped by means of symptom removal and symptom alleviation through direct suggestion and posthypnotic suggestion, but even more important is the application of hypnoanalysis in which the underlying problems are carefully investigated. The patient can often be regressed back to earlier levels of experience without much difficulty. The ability to better recall these disturbing and traumatic experiences can be very helpful in establishing etiologic facts.

I fully agree with Linderland Kroger that hypnoanalysis presents the possibility of helping greater numbers of patients by allowing access, more quickly, to the root causes of their problems. In most cases, a therapeutic transference can be established with the patient, often in several sessions that might otherwise take months or years. After all, the doctor must be concerned with helping the patient to communicate his problems in a meaningful and realistic manner, for without the establishment of therapeutic communications, psychotherapy is impossible. Under hypnosis, causal factors can often be fully explored and pinpointed. Hypnotherapy can be helpful as an adjunctive in the resolution of such conflicting patterns—reaction formations and defenses and in furthering gratifying and constructive affective and behavioral modification.

TREATMENT OF PREMENSTRUAL AND MENSTRUAL CONDITIONS

Since hypnosis can effectively relax smooth muscles, I have found that relaxation suggestion can often rapidly relieve premenstrual and menstrual cramps. The cramps and muscle tension are often caused by premenstrual anxiety. This anxiety can be rapidly allayed by hypnotherapy, i.e., Alice, a 25-year old married woman suffered from severe premenstrual and menstrual cramps and backache ever since she first began menstruating at 12. Her condition became progressively worse. She began to dread the onset of her menstrual cycle.

Under hypnosis she promptly revealed that she had heard her mother complain continuously about her cramps and backache. She could recall mother saying, "Someday you'll suffer like this, too, and you'll know what it means." As a consequence Alice built up quite a dread of menstruation. She recalls how tense, frightened and upset she was the first time. She recalled the cramps as well as her fear.

After consciously ventilating her recollections, pointing out that the fears were planted in her mind and that the condition was not organic, she felt much relieved. She came to realize that the psychological influence used in hypnosis could relieve her condition completely so that there could not be anything organically wrong. Reassurances that her anxiety, tension, cramps and backache would soon disappear completely just as they had in the trance proved most beneficial. Her condition was resolved rapidly and she has had no reoccurrence.

TREATMENT OF FUNCTIONAL GYNECOLOGICAL CONDITIONS

Hypnotherapy has proven to be of considerable value in functional gynecological conditions induced by emotional disturbances, such as amenorrhea, dysmenorrhea, menorrhagia, metorrhagia, pseudocyesis, pruritis vulvae and vaginae, vaginismus, frigidity, functional leucorrhea, sterility, and certain menopausal symptoms.

AMENORRHEA

Dunbar has pointed out that "in many cases, functional amenorrhea could be cured by one hypnotic session." For example, she points out that a patient had been suffering from amenorrhea for two and one-half years. Menses was induced by hypnosis and regulated to occur on the first day of each month, at 7:00 A.M. to last for three days. Other authors such as Heyer, Kroger and Freed have discussed this subject and have observed that hypnosis could not only relieve pain but also influence the menstrual cycle. As pointed out earlier, amenorrhea is often present in connection with pseudocyesis. A case in point is that of a female patient who was quite disturbed because, although she had had a miscarriage, four months earlier, she felt she was still pregnant, as she could perceive movement. Examination of the abdomen revealed no uterine enlargement; she had no breast milk; and the pregnancy tests were negative. Under hypnosis, this patient revealed that she felt quite emotionally disturbed and insecure due to the fact that she had discovered that her husband was carrying on an affair with another woman. She stated that she was in no state to have another child; she already had five, and with her husband carrying on as he was, she "couldn't even bear the thought."

In another case involving amenorrhea, the patient was suffering from a marked secondary anemia and was being treated for this condition. Under hypnosis she revealed that she had overheard a remark of her doctor to his nurse concerning her anemic condition, and that she became so agitated that she noted her menstrual cycle diminishing. She was particularly disturbed because it had been rather light in color, almost pink, and then had suddenly disappeared. It was obvious that this patient's apprehension, which had been considerably heightened by the remarks she had overheard, concerning the seriousness of her condition, had contributed to the functional amenorrhea. When she was given adequate antianemic medication and reassurance under hypnosis that her condition would clear up rapidly, and that she would begin to menstruate normally at the next period in her cycle, she responded very promptly.

Absense and irregularities of menstrual flow frequently occur as a result of emotional disturbances and are often highly amenable to hypnotherapy. Marked repressed anxiety, rage or guilt may often markedly affect the menstrual cycle. Such conditions vary in degree from complete cessation to very light and irregular menstrual flow.

A recent case was that of a 37-year old patient who had been referred to me by another physician for treatment of a severe periodic alcoholism and reactive depression. She gave a history of irregular, very light flow, having had several episodes of this type monthly. Further investigation of this patient under hypnosis revealed that she came from a very traumatic home situation. Her parents had separated when she was eleven due to her father's heavy drinking and emotional instability. She had been reared by a very rigid, domineering and overprotective mother who had been quite possessive of her and had not encouraged her social development. As a result of her mother's influence and the tragic experience of her parents' marriage, she had come to regard marriage with a considerable amount of fear and foreboding. Although quite an attractive person who had had numerous suitors and a number of marriage proposals, she had been unable to make a decision to marry. She was generally possessed by strong feelings of ambivalence and indecisiveness. Torn by her fears and the guilt she felt toward these men whom she felt she had let down, she began to have increasing feelings of unworthiness and depression. She sought escape by throwing herself actively into her work and by attending numerous social functions to which she had access because of her position. Although she met many men, she began increasingly to avoid intimate relationships. This patient as a result of several hypnotherapeutic sessions and a conscious ventilation of her fears and guilt feelings was able to achieve her normal menstrual cycle and flow within a two-month period.

Hypnoanalysis revealed that this patient, because of having been made fearfully aware of the painful experiences of her mother, unconsciously rejected the feminine role and sought in many ways to identify with men in pursuing an independent career and in seeking emotional and material autonomy from men. Unconsciously she permitted herself to become unattractive to men, overweight, somewhat slovenly in her dress, to cut her hair short, etc. She expressed the wish that she had been born a male for "what did women have to look forward to? Just look at my mother."

It is, of course, best in such cases to recommend that the patient undergo a longer period of individual or group psychotherapy. In some cases in which the emotional disturbances are less marked, it is often possible to obtain subjective improvement and to restore the normal flow by means of direct hypnotic suggestion or by a combination of hormonal medication, or placebo, plus hypnotic suggestion. The effects of various drugs and placebos may be markedly intensified as a result of hypnotic suggestion and excellent therapeutic results achieved.

PSEUDOCYESIS

In some instances a complete cessation of menstruation is associated with pseudocyesis, false pregnancy. Such patients are generally quite fearful of pregnancy. They often develop marked obsessive feelings, difficult to dislodge, that they are pregnant. Deutsch and Dunbar have expressed the view that certain of these patients may have an intense aggressive wish to be pregnant, or a marked ambivalence toward pregnancy. Such conditions can persist for years and in some instances these patients will go to "term" and experience "pseudo-labor" pains. In the treatment of such cases, it is important to establish whether the patient is sufficiently in touch with reality and possesses enough insight to permit her to accept the fact that she is not pregnant. It is necessary to make the patient understandingly aware of the unconscious motives that are responsible for her condition. It is advantageous to utilize hypnoanalysis to determine the etiology of her neurotic feelings about pregnancy and to resolve these. I have observed several cases in which feigned or hysterical pregnancy was used to try to pressure a man into marrying the patient.

FUNCTIONAL DYSMENORRHEA

Hypnotherapy may be of considerable benefit in the treatment of this disorder. However, it must be emphasized that there are frequent organic causes, such as uterine retroversion, inflammatory conditions, neoplasms, adhesions, small cervix with "pinhole" os, and other conditions, which may be responsible for pain and discomfort. Therefore, careful gynecological examination must be made before the diagnosis of functional dysmenorrhea is made.

Patients present a wide range of complaints, such as persistent backache, particularly during the premenstrual and menstrual period, feelings of pelvic pain, pressure and discomfort, general malaise, lassitude, irritability and depression. Often referred pain of an arthritic or neuralgic character is complained of. Such patients are generally high-strung, anxious individuals. Under hypnosis they reveal the dread with which they've regarded menstruation. Frequently they associate menstruation with being "unwell," "unclean," and as "a curse" with which women are afflicted. Investigation into their childhood and adolescent development reveals a failure on the part of the mother to explain the biological nature and purpose of menstruation and to the frequent suppression of any discussion of the subject, in some cases to paint a dismal and painful picture of the "curse."

A typical case is that of 43-year old married woman who complained of persistent premenstrual and menstrual cramps for years. She had taken numerous medications for her condition, but largely to no avail. It was of further interest that during these periods she would generally have excessive urinary frequency. Gynecological examinations repeatedly revealed no uterine displacement or abnormalities of any kind. The patient was of a tense, nervous, impatient disposition who stated that while in college she had suffered a nervous breakdown. For the first several years she had suffered from frigidity in her marriage and had felt emotionally insecure and inadequate in her role as a woman. She revealed that she had been reared as a foster child since she was orphaned early in life and had a foster brother who had teased and tormented her unmercifully during her childhood. Her foster parents had often been cruel to her, and she felt that they had strongly favored their biological son. She had early developed deep misgivings about accepting her feminine role. Her foster mother had never bothered to explain menstruation or how babies were born to her. She recalls how to her horror she for the first time saw blood dripping down her leg in school and how terribly embarrassed and frightened she felt, not being aware of the menstrual onset. She had always felt deeply insecure and somewhat rejected by her foster parents, and her feelings toward them were characterized by a marked ambivalence. Under hypnosis she was enabled to recall that her foster mother would always talk about how she swelled up before menstruation and became puffy. She would frequently take purgatives, such as Epsom Salts, to reduce the swelling. It is interesting that this patient for years had purged herself similarly prior to the menstrual period believing that this might relieve the dreaded symptoms. She stated that the swelling of her uterus not only caused her backache but pressure on her bladder, hence the urinary frequency. This patient proved to be highly suggestible and responded to direct suggestion plus placebos and was markedly relieved by the hypnotherapy. Since the basic cause of her condition was due to rather deep-seated developmental pathology, she was placed under psychotherapy and has made an excellent recovery.

FUNCTIONAL UTERINE BLEEDING

Here again it is of great importance to rule out organic pathology such as a possible neoplasm, fibroid tumor, miscarriage, etc. However, there are instances when disturbing emotional factors, such as severe physical or mental strain, shock, overfatigue, anxiety may precipitate heavy uterine bleeding. Observations of this type are not uncommon following natural disasters, war or serious accidents. We are familiar with instances of young brides who have been highly tense and keyed up to have found themselves embarrassed on their wedding night by the sudden onset of menstrual bleeding. On the other hand, it is not uncommon to observe heavy menstrual bleeding following a serious argument or lovers' quarrel. Although fear of pregnancy more often gives rise to amenorrhea, there are instances reported in which the same has given rise to functional bleeding.

I recall the case of a 30-year old female referred from the University Hospital Gynecological Clinic with a history of marked uterine bleeding in which the referring doctors had not been able to establish any cause. It was interesting that when the patient was put into a hypnotic trance, the bleeding began to markedly diminish. There is ample evidence that hypnotic suggestion can markedly reduce bleeding. She then revealed that she had been acutely upset just prior to the onset of the bleeding over the fact that her husband had gotten intoxicated on the job and was dismissed. She had considerable anxiety since she had four young children, it was very cold weather, and the oil company was threatening to shut off the fuel supply. The patient was assured under hypnosis that steps would be taken to see that the fuel supply was not cut off. This seemed to relieve considerable anxiety. Hypnotic influence was further employed to try to get this patient to bring in her husband for a consultation, which she did. This patient was then put into a trance at the Clinic, her husband brought in, and the session conducted in his presence. The patient ventilated her deep concerns about her husband's conduct, his drinking, her fears for the children and their general security. The husband was so impressed by the strong affective discharge that he was deeply concerned. Following this session, he agreed to undergo treatment for his alcoholic condition. Since the change in attitude on the part of the husband, there has been a general marked improvement in this patient's condition and the excessive bleeding has stopped. The husband was later hypnotized and the wife permitted to sit in while the husband poured out his hurt feelings, much of which were infantile. He protested about her lack of demonstrative affection and warmth—her failure to give him any recognition or praise. It was apparent that he needed some encouragement, particularly because of his strong feelings of inferiority. This experience afforded her much insight into how she might improve the marriage relationship. She realized that when her husband felt deprived, frustrated and angry that he drank in order to hurt her.

PRURITIS VULVAE AND VAGINAE

Generally this condition is associated with a persistent vaginal discharge and irritation. On occasion a skin condition, such as a dermatitis, pediculosis pubis, or a glycosuria, may be involved. Many patients who suffer from pruritis vulvae reveal tendencies toward excessive preoccupation, guilt and anxiety concerning masturbation. Generally, it suffices to help the patient gain conscious insight into the cause of their condition. In many instances, factors which have interfered with the patient's making a satisfactory sexual adjustment may be rapidly uncovered under hypnosis. Vaginal itching is more commonly encountered in nervous patients in middle age or beyond. Not infrequently tension and anxiety can result in vaginal dryness associated with pruritis. Hypnotherapy has been most effective in relieving this latter condition. The sources of emotional tension can often be readily explored and resolved. Hypnotic suggestion plus a soothing cortisone ointment may be a highly effective remedy.

FUNCTIONAL LEUCORRHEA

Where a pathogenic organism is not found responsible for the condition, such as a protozoan or fungus infection, it is well to keep in mind the possibility of a functional disorder. Marked vaginal secretion is generally precipitated by sexual excitement even without coitus. This condition responds well to hypnotherapy. That psychogenic factors play a very important role here was clearly demonstrated by Bunnemann who not only relieved such a case of a longstanding leucorrhea, but even provoked the condition experimentally, thus establishing without a doubt its psychogenic etiology.

With reference to the above condition, I recall a 35-year old woman who had been quite disturbed about a persisting vaginal discharge. Clinical checks revealed no infectious cause. Under hypnosis, this patient revealed that she was almost constantly obsessed with a desire for sexual intercourse. Although she stated that she had indulged in the same with innumerable men and had, because of her difficulty in attaining gratification, finally resorted to perverse methods of attaining orgasm, she still found herself generally ungratified. This nymphomanic condition was further explored under hypnosis, and as a result, this patient is now undergoing psychotherapy. Hypnotherapy was instrumental both in rapidly relieving the excessive discharge and in aiding this patient to understand the orginal causes of her condition and to overcome her vaginal frigidity.

Hypnoanalysis revealed severe neurotic conflicts about accepting the feminine role. There was marked identification with her father, penis envy, and a definite desire to be a man. She was very happy when she recalled under hypnosis the times she and her father had gone fishing and hunting together. She had always felt somewhat rejected and deprecated by her mother. Whenever she entered the kitchen and tried to help mother, it seemed that she could never satisfy her. When she helped father, on the other hand, she always got that pat on the back. Her brother always got the lion's share of the attention and privileges. She felt that she was penalized in being a girl. She revealed a marked masculine phallic character and a marked resistance toward assuming the passive, receptive, submissive feminine role. She had found herself repeatedly repelled by healthy, aggressive males and particularly drawn toward passive, neurotic ones whom she could control and dominate. As a result of hypnotherapy and analysis, the successful resolution of her problem was greatly accelerated.

FUNCTIONAL STERILITY

When a woman has not conceived over a longer period and after careful gynecological exploration, utilizing air tubal insufflation or lipoidal injection, no tubal obstruction or cervical displacement can be found and following examination of the husband to rule out the possibility of sterility, there is a considerable likelihood that we are dealing with a functional sterility. This condition appears to be on the basis of clinical observation more prevalent than had been hitherto supposed. It appears that emotional tensions (anxiety, rage) may lead to marked spasm of the Fallopian tubes so that passage and union of sperm and ovum cannot occur. Women who have not conceived over a period of years may develop marked anxiety and feelings of inadequacy. This leads to a secondary build-up of tension which can and often does apparently aggravate the preexisting condition. Fear of remaining childless may often assume the character of an obsession. Such a condition can also give rise to frigidity in the woman and may even produce symptoms of impotence in the husband. How often, in sheer desperation, a couple may decide to adopt a child only to find that several months later the wife is pregnant. It appears that the relaxation of tension often relieves the tubal spasms and makes conception possible. Hypnoanalysis of such cases reveals that at the root of the original tension may be such factors as aversion to sexuality, regarding it as "dirty," "immoral," "animalistic," "not for nice people," painful, etc. Such factors as fear of pregnancy and childbirth often prevail.

In a case of a 33-year old woman who had been married eleven years without conceiving and in which there was no evidence of any gynecological problem, she revealed the following under hypnosis: She was the only child, her parents were highly religious, leading citizens in a small town. She had always been supervised quite rigidly, was not permitted to play freely, and her associations with boys were strictly curtailed. Her mother had repeatedly warned her against the possibility that she might be taken advantage of, attacked, or abused by the opposite sex. This was particularly stressed because the patient had matured early and was unusually attractive. On one occasion, when she was 14, she was attacked and raped by a 16-year old boy on her way home from school. After this traumatic episode, her freedom was even more restricted. Under hypnosis she admitted that prior to the rape incident, she had acted teasing and seductive toward boys, although she appears to have been unaware of this at the time. Under hypnosis she further revealed her feelings that she regarded coitus as vulgar and unpleasant and that she frequently felt constriction of the vaginal muscles when her husband attempted to penetrate. There were times when his forceful attempts to penetrate were most painful and revolting. She had come to anticipate intercourse with a considerable amount of dread. With conscious ventilation of factors concerning her early rearing, her marked reaction to the traumatic experience of rape and the development of insight and awareness, her anxiety and tension markedly subsided. She was encouraged under hypnosis to accept group psychotherapy and has since made an excellent adjustment. Her condition of vaginismus was resolved, and she was able to look forward to sexual relations with pleasurable anticipation. Eight months after the onset of treatment, she became pregnant.

FRIGIDITY

Perhaps in no area of gynecological disorders has hypnotherapy proved of greater benefit than in the treatment of functional frigidity and impotence. The causes of frigidity are numerous. Among the most common are cases such as the aforementioned in which the patient suffered a severe traumatic experience with the opposite sex. A very common cause of frigidity is the fear of pregnancy. Very often the frigid patient reveals a history of experiencing disappointment or pain in her initial sexual experience and afterwards anticipates the same. Recently, a young woman of 28, a mother of three children, came to our clinic in a state of reactive depression stating that she had been frigid for several years and complained of marked nervous tension, irritability and insomnia. She was consciously unable to explain why she felt as she did. She was questioned closely about her marital life and her husband's attitude, but she did not communicate anything that might explain her condition. She was then put into a deep hypnotic trance and in her fantasy made to experience a coital relationship with her husband. She entered into the fantasy, reliving the experience quite intensely, and then suddenly cried out in a disturbed voice, "For heaven's sake, why do you have to bring up such things just at this time?" When pressed for an explanation, the patient stated, "He always manages to say something disturbing to me just when I am about to achieve the climax." Further elaboration of her husband's attitude toward her revealed evidence of sadistic traits. After conscious ventilation of this problem with the patient and her husband, it has been possible to resolve the problem.

In many instances, frigidity can be symptomatically relieved by putting the patient into a medium-to-deep trance and giving strong suggestion that she was going to be enabled to attain a very gratifying orgasm after taking a very powerful sexual stimulant which would have the effect of causing a most enjoyable climax. The patient would actually be given, in most instances, an herb-like liquid placebo, the effects of which would be explained in detail to the patient while in the trance. A strong anticipatory reaction of pleasure is thus created. In some instances, where it is felt indicated, a tablet placebo can be given.

The remarkable influence of suggestion in such conditions is illustrated by the following case of a 35-year old woman with five children who had been referred for hypnotherapy because of nicotinism. The patient came several hundred miles for treatment. She was most anxious because her physician had told her that she had a precancerous lesion in her throat. While under hypnosis she revealed that she had been frigid all of her married life. She was given the above suggestive therapy plus a sexual placebo. Ten days later she telephoned quite excitedly and overjoyed. She stated, "You haven't only cured me of smoking, doctor, but I've also become a real woman. I am so happy." She then explained that her husband had come home for a weekend and that she had attained eleven orgasms during that period. It has been six months since this communication. According to recent follow-up, this patient has continued her remarkable improvement. Gone are her feelings of inadequacy, nervousness and depression. It is important to point out here that the initial gains in this case have led to a general improvement in her marital and family life.

A 29-year old mother of six children came to the clinic in a very depressed, despondent state, suffering from hysteria, fatigue and marked nervousness. She spoke in a low anxious tone, and there was noticeable finger tremor and startle reaction. She had marked difficulty in communicating. She was relaxed without difficulty during the first session by my endogenic method. The trance was deepened by reverse counting technique and by hand levitation.

The patient was then able to communicate freely. Her immediate primary concern was her fear of conceiving another child. She felt very insecure in her marriage. She had become completely frigid in her marital relations following the discovery that her husband had apparently been having an affair with another woman. He had recently been very accusatory and irritable, projecting his own repressed guilt on to her. He had always tended to belittle and deprecate her generally. He was, she felt, almost impossible to satisfy. He made continuous excessive demands upon her. This continuous harangue had contributed to her growing lack of responsiveness to her husband. She repressed her feelings and was even fearful of openly accusing her husband, partly because she felt it might be too upsetting for the children and precipitate his leaving.

An attempt was made to contact the husband. He appeared quite resistive to coming in to discuss his wife's condition. He was finally prevailed upon to come in. On this occasion, the wife was hypnotized, and he sat through the session. Her deep feelings of hurt, humiliation, outrage, and anxiety poured out. During the session, it was possible to discuss the likelihood with her that he was projecting his own guilt (self-accusatory) feelings upon her by his repeated and unjustified accusations of infidelity, incompetence, etc. He was able to understand that his own mistreatment and deprecation of her had caused her to become increasingly frigid. It was that frigidity that had made him unreasonably resentful and frustrated, pushed him into seeking gratification elsewhere. At this time, he had been contemplating divorce. However, he had not yet taken the step because of his concern for the children.

After the husband had acquired a certain amount of insight into the situation, it was clearly pointed out that his wife could be helped to respond sexually, her anxiety concerning pregnancy could be alleviated by the use of proper contraception. It was further made evident to him that in order to save his family and help his wife, he would have to agree to fulfill the hopeful anticipation that could be instilled in his wife by hypnotic suggestion and that further disappointment and disillusionment would be seriously traumatic to his wife. Partly as a result of his newly acquired insights and due to his own reluctance to break up the family, the husband agreed to carry out his responsibilities in the matter.

Strong suggestion plus a sexual placebo, and a more considerate and demonstratively affectionate attitude on the part of the husband made it possible for the patient to rapidly overcome her frigidity.

MENOPAUSE

Treatment of menopausal conditions is an important area. In this connection, hypnotherapy can be of great benefit, particularly in the treatment of menopausal anxiety states, hysterical reactions, subjective discomfort, such as hot flashes, excessive sweating, conversion pain, fatigue, insomnia. The practitioner should of course be aware that many of these symptoms may actually be related to deeper conflicts of which the patient is unaware. These may range from disturbance at the thought of no longer being able to conceive a child or guilt over not having borne a child and having achieved fulfillment of the maternal drive, to fears of growing old and of death. Feelings of worthlessness and inadequacy are often associated with deeper guilt feelings which come to the fore during the menopausal period. It is therefore advisable to refer more deep-seated cases of this type for psychotherapy.

Of particular benefit to many patients suffering from menopausal disorders has been in our experience the combined use of hypnotic suggestion plus medication, such as placebos, hormones, sedatives, analgesics, etc. We have found that the effect of the drugs can be markedly potentiated by means of hypnotic suggestion. It is always better to try placebos first. As a result of the initial improvement generally achieved with such patients by the aforementioned method, they tend to revise their attitudes and feelings about the menopause.

This is borne out in the words of a patient, "Well, I'm not really finished after all. The change of life is not as bad as I thought it was." This patient had had the typical attitude of contemplating the menopause with considerable apprehension. She had heard so much talk about the change of life and how women suffer, and she had already resigned herself to going through a painful ordeal. When she realized that she still could feel young, vibrant and alive and could enjoy her marital relations, her attitude markedly changed.

Frequent menopausal tension and depression are often associated with excessive drinking, as in the following case: This was a 51-year old woman, the wife of a distinguished professional man, mother of several children, who was causing her husband marked embarrassment in the community by her periodic severe drinking. History revealed that the drinking had its onset when she first began to note a marked diminution of her menstrual flow, and experienced hot flashes. She was particularly troubled by nervous tension and insomnia. Although she had been only a social drinker previously, she reached out more and more for alcohol to relieve her tension and sleeplessness. She was treated at several clinics without success.

Under hypnosis, she complained that no one had been able to really understand her feelings and that furthermore she felt very insecure in her relationship to her husband, fearful of his rejection and disapproval. The husband was described as a critical, demanding person who had limited insight into his wife's and children's feelings. He was too occupied professionally to enter closely into their lives. As she stated, "When he was home, he was rather aloof and far away. Both I and the children continually sought reassurances of his love, interest, and companionship, but he remained largely shut in, withdrawn, and silent." She was first conditioned under hypnosis to an aversion to the taste and smell of alcoholic spirits by means of the endogenic technique, following which she was brought into individual psychotherapy. Both she and her husband were given group psychotherapy. The patient was given an imitation ovarian hormone preparation (actually a placebo) in combination with the hypnotic suggestion. Suggestion was further used to encourage her communication and rapport in psychotherapy. This patient responded beautifully and has remained abstinent now for four years. Her entire attitude has changed, and she feels that the life to the family as a whole is much happier due to the increased understanding and insight gained by her husband as well as herself.

Another case is that of a 56-year old woman who had also resorted to alcohol as an escape from her menopausal symptoms. She had complained primarily of hot flashes, marked nervous tension, and insomnia, and of being so irritable that she found it difficult to get along with coworkers on the job. Her anxiety and tension had been markedly accentuated following her husband's death eight years earlier. Prior to his death, she stated that she had only drunk socially and never been intoxicated. In defending her drinking, she stated, "What can I do? I feel so miserable, so alone, and who would want me, I am 56-years old." The patient stated that whenever she felt upset, she felt an immediate compulsion to drink, at times struggling with herself but unable to resist the crutch which gave her some relief but caused such disagreeable hangovers. She was given the hypnotic aversion treatment during which she developed intense nausea but no emesis. She stated that actually after drinking, she would get thoroughly nauseated during the hangover but rarely vomited. This patient responded remarkably well to a combination of Stelazine, two mgs. b.i.d., which was potentiated by hypnotic suggestion. She is getting along splendidly and has now been completely abstinent for over a year.

In many instances, it was possible, as in the first case mentioned, to rapidly aid the husband in gaining insight into his wife's disturbed feelings by having him sit through a session in which she discharged her hurt and anxious feelings in his presence. There is little doubt that the abreaction in his presence was beneficial to her as well.

PREOPERATIVE ANXIETY

Hypnosis can be most helpful in relieving preoperative anxiety, as in the following instance of a 45-year old woman who had to undergo a hysterectomy. Her anxiety was so great that her gynecologist referred her for help. She was not only fearful of the operation but also at the thought of losing her uterus, the fear that she would no longer be a complete woman, and anxiety that her husband would reject her. Her anxiety concerning the operation itself was most acute. She was hypnotized without difficulty and then trained in autohypnosis. In a short time she was able to relax herself into a hypnotic trance quite rapidly using the endogenic method. The procedure was discussed with her gynecologist, and she relaxed herself approximately two hours before surgery and did not experience any trauma or discomfort whatsoever. As a result of her hypnotic relaxation, the surgeon advised me that she required far less anaesthetic and her recovery was rapid.

As stated previously, hypnosis can be of considerable value for purposes of inducing hypnoanalgesia and anaesthesia. This is possible in a large percentage of the cases. The procedure is quite useful in minor surgical procedures, such as dilatation and curetage, cervical cauterization, etc. Hypnoanaesthesia may be used in major surgical procedures although it is best used in combination with general anaesthesia, greatly reducing the anaesthetic requirement, thus reducing the toxicity and facilitating recovery of the patient.

GYNECOLOGICAL EXAMINATION

There are instances in which patients show considerable resistance or anxiety regarding pelvic examinations. We had one such patient at the clinic who had been having irregular excessive bleeding and had for months refused to undergo a pelvic examination. The examination was greatly facilitated by the marked relaxation of the abdominal, vaginal and pelvic muscles. Her gynecologist consulted on the matter. The patient was easily relaxed into a hypnotic trance and the pelvic examination carried out. The patient was given a posthypnotic suggestion that she would no longer have anxiety about pelvic examinations, that there was no reason for this anxiety, since she had not experienced any discomfort whatsoever. The patient thereafter readily submitted to examination.

OPHTHALMOLOGY

The value of hypnosis in ophthalmology should not be underestimated. For many patients, and particularly children, treatment of the eyes understandably involves considerable anxiety. This apprehension can often be readily allayed by hypnosis. Another problem which presents difficulties for the ophthalmologist is that of immobilizing the apprehensive patient so that treatment may be facilitated. As a result of hypnosis the patient can not only be relieved of anxiety but can remain immobilized in one position— most important, the fixation of the eyes can be obtained and treatment greatly facilitated. In addition, pain and discomfort can be relieved by means of hypnosis. Hypnosis presents an ideal method for preoperative and pretreatment relaxation of the patient, after which cocaine and other medications can be instilled in the eye and the patient spared the usual sufferings of preoperative tension. This is of especially great importance in such types of eye surgery as retinal detachment and cataract surgery where the mental as well as physical relaxation of the patient may be of paramount importance. Furthermore, it is significant that the effect of cocaine as an anaesthetic can be potentiated considerably by inducing a preanaesthetic hypnotic analgesia.

Hypnosis can be of great value in differential diagnosis, particularly in differentiating functional and hysterical eye conditions such as hysterical blindness or hysterical eye pain, etc. Hysterical blindness, of course, is generally of the telescopic type, although certain variations of hysterical blindness occur. Generally, there is no difficulty in differentiating hysterical blindness due to the fact that it is usually bilateral and the patient usually has a circular constricted field of vision. The value of hypnosis in the treatment of ocular headache is very significant. In most cases prompt relief of such headaches can be obtained by means of hypnosis. I recall a physician who himself had suffered from severe migraine type of headaches which started with ocular pain. He had not responded well to analgesics, and when hypnosis was attempted, he was promptly relieved of his pain. It was then suggested that he could relieve himself of his pain, whenever he felt that an attack was coming on, by self-hypnosis. The patient was given the necessary instructions and training in autohypnosis. Following this treatment episode, the patient was not seen for approximately one year, at which time he stated that he had never had a recurring headache after the initial treatment. He then went on to explain that after he had realized that his ocular headache could be relieved by means of hypnosis, he lost his apprehension and never had another headache. His apprehension was particularly relieved because he knew how to prevent another attack from occurring.

Hypnosis is, of course, of great value in the treatment of emotionally based eye disorders such as eye tics, blinking, squinting, and so forth. By means of hypnosis one may often rapidly uncover the neurotic defensive mechanism involved. Further psychotherapy can then be instituted to help the patient overcome his trouble.

The importance of hypnosis for both preoperative and postoperative treatment in many conditions such as cataract operations for the relief of pain, tension, and anxiety which often occur in such patients is significant. Rest can be facilitated in many instances by means of hypnosis. Hypnosis can be of value in reducing inflammation and swelling through its antiphlogistic effect. The importance of hypnosis for postoperative or followup treatment is significant. A patient cannot only be relieved of suffering, but can be strongly encouraged to cooperate with the treatment regime. This is particularly true with the longer term treatment of strabismus and eye muscle weakness where corrective exercises are necessary. Of special value is the application of hypnotic and posthypnotic suggestion in cases in which there is considerable resistance to such corrective treatment and exercises.

Hypnosis can also be of value in getting patients adjusted to wearing glasses. One area where it is helpful is in training patients in the ability to tolerate contact lenses. This has presented considerable difficulty to many ophthalmologists during the early stages when patients are becoming accustomed to wearing lenses. Hypnotic suggestion can be utilized to reduce corneal sensitivity.

We have also found that hypnosis is valuable in running controlled responses for refraction, that often refraction difficulties could be uncovered under hypnosis which were not consciously apparent, particularly if the refraction was of a functional or hysterical type. In some instances hypnosis can be of value in evaluating patient's color responses that may be consciously masked, particularly in patients with borderline color blindness.

It should be noted that where prolonged work on the eyes, such as prolonged refraction testing and eye examination are required, which is often tiring for patients, hypnosis can greatly relieve the strain and make the patient more comfortable. Furthermore, when it is necessary for the patient to take medication regularly and instill drops, as in glaucoma, particularly in those cases where the patient is somewhat negligent or uncooperative, hypnosis can be an important factor in securing regular cooperation. I have also used hypnosis to relax patients with interocular hemorrhage as well as inflammatory eye conditions. The cooperation of patients during treatment procedures may be greatly enhanced by hypnosis.

HYPNOSIS IN THE SPECIALTIES: EAR-NOSE-THROAT

In ear, nose and throat work, hypnosis has marked value and can be frequently utilized to relieve such disturbing symptoms as anxiety, pain, and particularly the apprehension which most patients feel for the otolaryngologist. Again, hypnosis is an ideal tool for relieving tension and anxiety in children, since this often presents a problem. There are in ear, nose and throat work of course, many minor surgical procedures that are employed, and it is here that hypnotic analgesia can be very effectively used; for example, in the treatment of sinus or nasal conditions, etc. where repeated treatment is necessary. After the initial induction when hypnotic analgesia is attained, it is very easy to bring about subsequent hypnotic analgesia and to conduct further follow-up treatment in this manner, relieving both pain and apprehension in the patient. Also hypnosis can help to potentiate any surface anaesthetic or local anaesthetic used for the relief of pain. Hypnosis is also of value, not only in the preoperative preparation for relief of anxiety but for the motor relaxation of the patient, making him a better operative subject. Bleeding and inflammation can also be reduced by hypnotic suggestion.

In those patients where ear, nose and throat work produces gagging, nausea, vomiting, etc., hypnosis can be a valuable tool in relieving this, so that the patient can be treated more easily and less traumatically. Hypnosis can be very valuable in the postoperative relief of pain and discomfort, and to aid the patient to rest and relax. Furthermore, it is very important in securing the cooperation of the patient in complying with the doctor's orders in the treatment regime.

Hypnosis can be used also for purposes of differential diagnosis where there are feelings of pain or pressure which are not of organic origin. Posthypnotic suggestion can be used with eye, ear, nose and throat patients very effectively to further their relaxation, relief of pain after treatment and rest after operative procedures. I have been instructing ear, nose, throat specialists in treating smokers since they felt that smoking was contributory to sinus, nose, throat and bronchial problems.

HYPNOSIS IN OTHER SPECIALTIES: ORTHOPEDICS

In orthopedics, of course, the acute trauma, swelling, and pain of the patient may be severe. The emotional trauma is often considerable as well. The patient has generally been exposed to an acute accident. Not only pain, of course, but apprehension can be relieved, and the induction of rest facilitated through hypnosis. Hypnosis is excellent for this purpose, especially if combined with local or general anaesthetic or hypnotic sedative drugs. It will potentiate the effects of all of these and the patient may require less anaesthetic or drugs. Hypnosis can be of great value with those cases that have to wear casts or assume uncomfortable positions, immobilized for long periods of time. It has been found that not only hypnosis, but as noted earlier, in many cases teaching the patient to relax by means of autohypnosis can be of great value in relieving the patient and in facilitating nursing care.

The relaxation of patients who have been in traumatic accidents and in particular of children is of great importance, and here hypnosis often can be of great benefit. Often, patients having to wear casts and to maintain uncomfortable fixed positions for prolonged periods have difficulty in resting. Hypnosis and autohypnosis can be useful here. Hypnosis can also be used to reduce bleeding, particularly where there have been open reductions and operative orthopedic procedures performed. One area in which hypnosis has proven to be of great value in orthopedic work is in retraining patients to wear prosthetics and artificial limbs, and also, of course, in reactivating and exercising limbs that have been immobilized for long periods of time. I have had a number of cases where hypnosis was helpful in retraining patients to walk again after having been immobilized in pelvic casts, etc., for long periods of time. Hypnosis can do a great deal to help the patient regain confidence in the use of his extremities, in coordination and balance.

The value of hypnosis in reducing edema or inflammation is significant. Hypnosis can also be of value after cast removal and prolonged immobilization in manual-manipulating of joints or extremities. Furthermore, hypnosis as aforementioned is also of value in differential diagnosis where there is physical impairment of the extremities of a hysterical functional type.

HYPNOSIS IN THE OTHER SPECIALTIES: UROLOGY

Genitourinary Conditions

In urology, hypnosis can be of great value in relieving the pain, suffering, and discomfort of patients. I have encouraged its use extensively for catheterization of patients and for minor procedures. It is of considerable value in preoperative preparation of the patient, and can be used in the dilation of strictures, and cystoscopic examination, not only in relieving pain, but in immobilizing the patient. It is also valuable in relieving apprehension in these patients, particularly in preparation for major surgery, relaxing their tension, and sparing them considerable trauma. In many cases, it is of real value in postoperative care in furthering the relief of pain and discomfort.

The importance of relieving intractable pain in cancer patients where there is involvement of the genitourinary tract must not be overlooked. Patients can often not only be relieved of this pain, but can be trained in many instances to relieve themselves by means of autohypnosis. Furthermore, the effects of analgesic drugs can be potentiated by means of hypnosis. The value of hypnosis in genitourinary work for differential diagnosis where there is a problem of differentiating hysterical conditions from organic conditions is significant. In many conditions such as a functional polyurea, the frequency can be relieved and the cause usually readily determined. Psychogenic urethral, bladder and prostatic pain can be readily relieved and explored.

As was discussed earlier, the treatment of impotence by means of hypnosis has also been quite successful. The relief of both physical pain and psychic trauma in the treatment of priapism and phymosis has been achieved by hypnosis.

I have found that hypnotic suggestion is helpful in the treatment of priapism. The procedure which I employed was to combine such with venus puncture and withdrawal of blood up to approximately 1,000 ccs. within 24 to 48 hours. Frequently, simply the introduction of a needle into a vein plus hypnotic suggestion is alone sufficient to relieve priapism.

In summary, hypnosis is of particular value in the treatment of functional urologic disorders such as polyuria, impotence, priapism, pseudogonorrhea. It can be of value, too, in catheterization—pyelograms; for preoperative relaxation; for postoperative care; to further cooperation with regard to dietary regimen, fluid intake, the taking of medication, and coming in for treatment. In addition, hypnosis can be employed effectively to relieve pain, burning and discomfort, to influence patient to accept surgery or treatment which is definitely indicated.

In some instances of urinary bladder distension and difficulty in urinating because of sphincter closure, it is often possible to relax the sphincter by means of hypnotic suggestion.

DERMATOLOGY

There are a considerable number of skin disorders in which psychological factors play either an important primary or secondary role. In those instances where emotional disturbances are in the foreground, hypnotherapy can be of great benefit. Furthermore, it is well to keep in mind that hypnosis can be effectively employed as an adjuvant to treatment because it frequently provides a ready means to relieve the subjective suffering of the patient, symptoms of itching, burning, and pain. Also, because of its remarkable antiphlogistic action, hypnosis can often rapidly relieve or ameliorate swelling, redness, edema, and psychic disturbing symptoms such as restlessness, insomnia, etc.

TREATMENT OF INFLAMMATORY SKIN REACTIONS

The marked antiinflammatory effect which can be produced through hypnosis is illustrated by the following case, first observed in 1949, and which I reported together with photographic illustrations of the lesions and the changes in 1952 to the Section on Neurology and Psychiatry, District of Columbia Medical Society. A 42-year old male, an abstinent morphine addict (a hospitalized case which could be properly controlled) complained of burning and itching in a localized area in the left gluteal region. This burning and itching was refractory to ordinary medication. He was treated by means of a placebo plus hypnotic suggestion, whereupon the condition promptly subsided. An attempt was then made to experimentally provocate the skin reaction again by means of hypnotic suggestion plus placebo. In approximately 72 hours the patient developed a full-blown picture of herpes Zoster neuritis with pain radiating to the areas of the respective spinal ganglion. The patient had the typical herpes vesicles and the discomfort due to the inflammatory and radiating pain was marked. Again, the previous procedure for relieving the condition was applied, placebo plus hypnotic suggestion, and again there was a remission. The condition was again provocated, after several days' interval, and again a remission induced. It was unmistakably clear that in this instance a herpes zoster neuritis and ganglionitis could be both provocated and relieved by means of hypnotic suggestion. As a result of these observations, I concluded that since it was possible to provocate an inflammatory reaction by means of hypnotic suggestion, it should also be possible to relieve inflammation by the same means.

As previously noted, Forel in Switzerland had earlier reported the production of burn blisters by means of hypnotic suggestion. His work stimulated further research, and in 1938 Helig and Hoff reported that they could produce typical herpes simplex lesions by means of hypnotic suggestion in proven herpes virus carriers. These investigators found that they could not produce lesions by merely suggesting to the patient that he was experiencing itching; however, when they gave strong suggestions that the patient was experiencing a very unpleasant emotionally disturbing situation, the herpes lesions developed. Certainly such effects could not be produced in every patient but were most apparent in those patients who were not only highly prone to suggestive influence, but who also revealed a deeply disturbed emotional background, and as a result were in a state of hyperaffectivity. In my opinion, such patients have highly sensitive vasomotor response. Since the degree of hyperaffectivity is generally highly increased during the hypnotic trance, such marked reactions as the above can occur. Certainly such clinical and experimental evidence clearly reveals the definite cause and effect interrelation between mind and body.

Another illustration of this link between mind and body is that of a 38-year old female physician I observed suffering from a severe thrombophlebitis due to markedly inflamed varicosities of the right lower extremity. The referring physician had advised that the patient had great difficulty in resting because she was very uncomfortable, with her leg constantly in an elevated position. The patient's anxiety and pain were marked. She was relaxed promptly by the endogenic method and a prolonged hypnotic sleep was induced. Prior to the induction of the sleep, she was given strong direct suggestions that the inflammation in her leg was going to subside rapidly and that she would feel relieved of pain and discomfort upon awakening. She was kept in the deep relaxation approximately 72 hours with the exception of several brief intervals for feeding. Following this period, there was a remarkable reduction in inflammation, and the patient showed an overall general improvement. In fact, no less than 48 hours following the hypnotic sleep, her condition was so much improved that the elevated leg splint which was causing her such discomfort could be removed.

DERMATOLOGY: COMBINED TREATMENT

Hypnosis is particularly valuable in the management of those skin disorders in which it is so often necessary to obtain the cooperation of the patient in the treatment regime. All too often, patients irritate their own skin lesions by scratching, causing secondary aggravation and infection. The problem, further, of holding the patient to a specific therapeutic regime which often includes topical application, proper physiotherapy, diet and rest often poses difficulties for the physician. Hypnotic suggestion can be very helpful in securing such cooperation. The following is an example of the particular value of the combined use of medication plus hypnotic suggestion.

A 70-year old male patient complained of a very severe generalized itching dermatitis, more marked over the back and abdomen. The patient had been previously treated by a physician for two weeks unsuccessfully; in spite of the starch baths prescribed, the skin became more inflamed, the itching more severe, and the condition, on the whole, more aggravated. The impression was that of an acute dermatitis apparently due to some external toxic factor. The patient suffered extreme discomfort and anxiety, and had great difficulty in resting properly, since he spent most of the night scratching himself. Investigation brought up the fact that the bed sheets and underclothes of the patient had been washed with a strong detergent soap which his wife had employed for the first time. A dermal patch test revealed that he was highly sensitive to this agent. As a first step in clearing up his condition, the use of a neutral, bland soap, instead, was ordered. During the hypnotic trance, the patient was given direct suggestion and assurance that since the cause of his irritation was now known and removed, he would rapidly get well, his itching and inflammation would cease, and his skin condition would clear up altogether in a short time. Further, it was suggested that because of the marked symptomatic improvement, he would be able to sleep well and rest comfortably. The patient made a very rapid and uneventful recovery, and had no further difficulty in resting.

In many instances, suggestive hypnotherapeutic influence can be markedly accentuated by supplementing with infra-red, ultra-violet or light dermal doses of X-ray while the patient is in the hypnotic trance, or by utilizing posthypnotic suggestion with administration of physical therapy following the trance.

DERMATOLOGY: TREATMENT OF PSYCHOSOMATIC SKIN DISORDERS

A very lovely girl of 28, married, who had been a beauty queen and had always been quite conscious of her attractiveness presented herself with a problem of a compulsion to tear at her skin, which she failed to consciously control. As a result, the patient had numerous scars around her face and neck. Background history revealed that she had had a very domineering, severe mother and a weak father, and that her mother had been very strict and had greatly limited her social life. She had felt this restriction particularly keenly through her teens when, because of the restrictions imposed by her mother, she was unable to participate in social functions with her friends. Further, her mother had succeeded in making her feel very guilty at protesting the treatment she received, and had fostered a guilt ridden and dependent attitude in her. The father, never having successfully opposed the mother, did not object to the maltreatment she received at the hands of the mother. She had built up a constantly increasing amount of repressed hostility towards her mother and had reacted similarly towards her husband. As a result of this inability to externalize her deep resentment, she unconsciously turned it inward and began to tear at her skin. A further study of this case in subsequent hypnotic session revealed a deep-seated masochistic tendency in which she unconsciously sought attention, sympathy and love through self-injury. Interestingly, she married a man who had obvious sadistic traits and who himself unconsciously played on her masochism by repeatedly hurting her. She had great difficulty in discharging anger or rage thus engendered, and would, in her helpless, impotent rage, turn this destructive effect against herself. It was at these times that she felt like clawing at her skin. In this case hypnosis played an invaluable role in getting at the basic underlying causes of the patient's skin condition, and in helping her and her husband to acquire insight and eventually to achieve a resolution of their difficulties.

Strong emotional reactions such as anxiety, shame, self-consciousness are frequently precipitated by skin conditions. Many patients are very sensitive about skin lesions appearing on the face or visible parts of the body, while others may be extremely self-conscious due to the continual urge to scratch. Hypnosis, as indicated, is very helpful in relieving such discomfort and tenseness.

Hypnotherapy is of particular value in the treatment of skin conditions in which an excessive secretion or vasodilation occurs, e.g., hyperhidrosis, excessive oil secretion, seborrhea, and urticaria. There is now considerable experimental evidence of neurohormonal mechanisms, producing histamine and histamine-like substances which accumulate in the skin following emotional reactions resulting in vasodilation, sweating and even inflammatory reactions of the skin of varying degrees. Of note, further, is the vasoconstrictive effect of the skin and the scalp resulting from anxiety reactions. Vasoconstriction may contribute to excessive drying of the skin and scalp, and to poor oil secretion, contributing to hair loss. A case in point is that of a 32-year old woman who presented a disseminated type of hair loss. This type of distribution of hair loss is often linked with emotional etiology. The patient was pale, tense, and anxious; there was marked vasoconstriction. Her scalp was rather dry, with fine scaling apparent. Under hypnosis, the patient revealed that approximately a year earlier she had discovered evidence that her husband was involved with other women. The patient felt deeply insecure and threatened by this. Her concern over the future of her four children intensified these feelings. She revealed that she had been frigid since the birth of her last child and that her husband had become increasingly dissatisfied with the marital relationship. During the terminal months of her last pregnancy, he became involved with other women, often remaining away overnight. As a result, she grew despondent, apathetic and lost her drive and initiative. Psychotherapy and counseling on a conscious level resolved her frigidity and the marital relationship improved. As the patient's apprehension dimished, the hair loss gradually stopped.

Since the innervation of the skin and the scalp to a large extent is controlled by the automonic nervous system, it is clear that emotional factors can play a very important role in many disturbances in those areas. There is ample experimental evidence that urticarial lesions, localized edema and swelling, inflammation, blisters and even spontaneous localized hemorrhage have been treated successfully in this manner. There is as yet insufficient data to explain the fact that patients show very little dermal capillary or tissue bleeding under hypnotic suggestion. This is particularly marked if the patient is sufficiently deep so that hypnoanalgesia or anaesthesia exists. It is further interesting that by means of hypnotic suggestion, it is possible to create not only anaesthesia but hyperesthesia of the skin, and that patients can be made to experience various sensations such as paraesthesia, itching, tingling, pain, sensitivity to heat or cold, feelings of pleasure, etc. It is my opinion that these effects are as a result of central psychic changes causing selective alterations in the perception of stimuli coming from the body surface.

INDICATIONS FOR HYPNOTHERAPY IN DERMATOLOGICAL DISORDERS

As illustrated previously, the application of hypnosis for the relief of pain and itching has been quite successful in many cases. A great variety of skin conditions in which inflammation, pain, itching, and skin lesions are present may be markedly improved by hypnotherapy. Foremost among these are Urticarial Reactions, Erythrodermea, Hyper Hydrosis, Neurodermatitis, (Darier), Lichen Ruber Planus Verrucae, certain forms of Eczema, Pityrias Rosea, Contact Dermatitis, some types of Alopecia, and as aforementioned, Herpes Simplex and Zoster. Conditions which respond, but to a lesser degree, are Pemphigus Vulgaris, Acne Rosacea, Psoriasis, Spontaneous Hemorrhage, etc.

There are and always will be sceptics, and indeed, some of our colleagues are hard to convince; however, there are certain common skin reactions such as blushing, pallor, sweating, "goose pimples," which even lay people associate with such emotional reactions as anxiety, shame, rage, etc. For a long time, pediatricians have removed warts in children by the use of merely wakeful suggestion, i.e., painting the wart with a harmless dye and directly suggesting that it will soon disappear. This certainly supports the fact that Hyperkeratosis and certain cellular and benign neoplastic growth-stimulating effects may result from psychic emotional causes. Certainly, peptic ulcer is closely correlated with deep-seated emotional disturbances and a high percentage of peptic ulcer conditions are later complicated by gastric carcinoma.

It is well to emphasize, at this point, the significance of the use of hypnosis in ventilating and relieving pent-up states of tension in the form of abreaction in the treatment of many skin disorders. The authors observed the rapid resolution of skin conditions, not only after such catharsis occurred, but also when prolonged hypnotic sleep was induced, for varying periods of from two to seven days. Hypnotic suggestion can be indirectly quite successfully applied in many instances in conjunction with physiotherapy such as sun lamps, both ultra violet and infra red, and light dermal dosage of Bucky Rays. Of course, the physician can under hypnosis create hallucinations that the patient is being radiated, bathed, or otherwise treated with very beneficial results by direct suggestion.

Some authorities have recommended the use of direct suggestion in an attempt to remove disturbed attitudes underlying the skin condition. This can be done, but it is unwise to attempt it if the physician is not aware of the underlying psychopathology and is not equipped to deal with the problems arising; it would be wiser to refer such cases to a qualified, experienced psychiatrist.

In the treatment of the more chronic, refractory skin conditions, such as certain eczemas, psoriasis, it is important to keep in mind that the hypnotic suggestions given the patient should be of a character to convey reassurance and hopeful anticipation, thus allaying apprehension and despair. Certainly in these conditions it is of the utmost importance to explore the patient's concomitant, more deep-seated emotional conflicts and to resolve these. It is further highly important not to offer direct hypnotic suggestions implying that the condition will immediately clear up, or to raise false hopes, since such would only disillusion and undermine the patient's confidence in the physician. Rather, suggestions should be offered that the condition will improve gradually from day to day, and will ultimately clear up entirely. Further, suggestions should be given the patient to make him feel that he can do much in the way of cooperating with the treatment regime, diet, medication, etc., which will accelerate recovery, and that this cooperation is highly essential. Thus, the physician leaves himself a way out should the patient resist treatment and transfer the blame to the physician.

In summation, it should be stressed that hypnosis provides a most valuable adjunctive technique in the treatment of many dermatological disorders, not only for symptomatic relief of very disturbing characteristics, but also in the resolution of the underlying, more deep-seated emotional problems which are frequently involved in skin disorders. In no area of medicine is this close correlation between mind and body as well demonstrated as in the skin disorders. The application of combined methods employing hypnosis in conjunction with therapeutic agents for the treatment of skin conditions is highly promising. Much research is still needed in the field, particularly as related to the question of the influence of hypnotic suggestion on inflammatory reactions. There appears to be a close correlation also between hypnotic influence and skin manifestations of an allergic type, and this area also requires further investigation. There is no doubt that the effects of therapeutic agents in skin disorders can be potentiated by hypnotic suggestion.

NEUROLOGY

Hypnosis can be an invaluable aid in differential diagnosis in neurological conditions. Of interest in this connection is the case of a 46-year old business executive who was obsessed with the idea that he had a brain tumor. He went to a leading neurologist who was frankly baffled by his symptoms. He presented the classical clinical picture of a cerebellar pontive angle tumor. He complained of dizziness, headache, falling toward the right side and drifting toward the right when walking. He had been reading about this condition in a neurology book and became very panicked about his state. He could hardly function at work and became increasingly despondent, entertaining suicidal ideas.

He was put under hypnosis and given the suggestion that he could and would walk straight without falling to one side. Under hypnosis he walked a straight line on command. While still under hypnosis he was told to observe the fact that he could walk normally. In the trance he revealed the following: His onset of symptoms had developed shortly after a particular family tragedy. His older sister was seriously injured in an automobile accident. He was asked to go to Chicago to arrange for a neurosurgeon to operate on her which he did. Unfortuanately, the operation was not too successful, and his sister retained certain incapacities. His sister blamed him for the choice of the surgeon. This sister had always been very critical of B. and had tended frequently to make him feel guilty. Interestingly, B. had unconsciously incorporated her identical symptoms as a form of self-punishment. When the cause of his condition was explained, his symptoms began to rapidly clear up.

HYPNOSIS IN DENTISTRY

Hypnosis has already proven to be of significant value in the practice of dentistry, particularly in alleviating anxiety, pain and discomfort. My endogenic method is very rapid and effective for this purpose. Suggestions can be given when the patient is in a trance that he will experience a comfortable, pleasant, increasing numbness in his mouth and this pleasant numbness will be greatest in the gums. Further, the patient is given the suggestion that when he feels the needle, he will feel that side of his mouth growing numb and anaesthetic, that each time he feels the needle or the instrument, the area will feel increasingly numb and painless, and that soon he will only be able to feel a pleasant contact but no pain, no pain whatsoever.

Hypnosis can often be employed in suitable subjects without any anaesthetic. Generally, it is beneficial to combine hypnosis with a small or moderate amount of anaesthetic, i.e., a topical anaesthetic can be applied and suggestion given. Hypnosis can be employed to relieve anxiety and discomfort prior to and during the drilling of cavities, extractions or the fitting of bridges, crowns, dentures, etc. Hypnotic suggestion can be used to motivate patients to cooperate with instructions such as eating proper foods following treatment—oral hygiene, etc. Relief of pain can range from complete to partial hypnoanalgesia and anaesthesia. In oral surgery, the patient can be spared much of the preoperative dread and can be put in a much more cooperative and comfortable state of mind. Hypnosis can be of considerable value in relieving discomfort in orthodontic work. It can be of great value in dentistry with children, who often respond well to hypnosis and hypnotic suggestion.

Since under hypnosis, the patient is very compliant, hypnotic suggestion can be very helpful in securing excellent cooperation.

Chapter 9

HYPNOAVERSION THERAPY

Treatment of Chronic Alcoholism by Hypnotic Aversion

About 25 years ago I began to experiment with inducing Pavlovian conditioned reflexes under hypnosis. To my surprise, I found that associative conditioned responses could be established very rapidly in the hypnotic state. In fact, such conditioned responses could be established in some instances in one to three sessions. This was, of course, in sharp contrast to the long periods required to condition animals and humans by the conscious Pavlovian method.

I speculated on the possibility that this kind of conditioning might be of benefit to alcoholics. The problem was how to establish an effective aversive reaction so that the alcoholic, for example, would not only lose his desire for alcoholic beverages, but would become severely nauseated if he tried to drink.

I knew of the conscious conditioning used by Voegtlin, LeMere and others. However, I found such conscious conditioning to be both disturbing to the patient and frequently ineffective. Attempts to turn alcoholics against alcohol by direct hypnotic suggestion had also proven for the most part ineffective. The use of improvised fantasy aversion had likewise proven largely ineffective.

As a result of studying hypnotic regression, I had observed that an individual can vividly relive those past traumas which he personally had experienced at previous times in his life (phenomena of revivification). In the hypnotic state, the time sense is largely lost so that past and present can be closely correlated and associated as though occurring in the "here and now."

Hypnosis not only facilitates recall but can markedly potentiate both affective and past psychophysiological reactions as though they were actually occurring—this, while one is holding whiskey under the patient's nose or placing a cigarette in his mouth.

Very often the aversion reaction and the reliving of the past traumatic, disgust experience occurs after only one to two sessions. This conditioned response is then intensified with subsequent treatments. Normally within several sessions, the individual is able to relive the original, revolting, nauseous experience every time he tastes or smells the harmful substance, i.e., alcohol, cigarettes, high caloric food, etc. This reaction soon becomes reflexly automatic.

It must be emphasized that an induced fantasy experience does not evoke the intense and lasting, nauseant reaction that occurs when a former revolting life trauma is relived.

I continued experimenting with various methods in an attempt to create a lasting aversion to alcoholic spirits by means of hypnosis. Since the smell and taste of whiskey, beer, and wine are generally pleasurable to the alcoholic, I felt that it was necessary to attempt to create an aversion to the taste, smell, and thought of alcoholic beverages and, furthermore, that if the generally pleasant anticipatory reaction of the alcoholic to alcoholic beverages could be altered to one of disgust and displeasure, it would discourage any primary desire for drink. As mentioned, in my initial attempts I found that the aversion reactions could be intensified by having patients regress and relive the unpleasant "hangover" effects of alcohol in the hypnotic trance. In other words, under hypnosis the patient can relive his most disagreeable "hangover" intrapsychically, without having to ingest alcohol or nauseant drugs.

The basic rationale behind the hypnoaversion treatment procedure was that of Freud's pleasure principle and the efforts of the unconscious mind to evade or avoid reliving a painful, disgusting, or disagreeable experience. Then, too, Pavlov had demonstrated how conditioned reflexes and associative reactions could be established and how reactivity could be so intensified that a light stimulus would produce a marked response. It was hypothesized by Pavlov, Bechterew and Salter that the phenomenon of hypnosis resembled a conditioned response in that the subject becomes increasingly susceptible to hypnotic induction (phenomenon of "dressage"). Thus, it appeared similarly possible to "sensitize" and accelerate the development of conditioned reflex response by means of hypnosis. After brief conditioning even a slight whiff or taste of alcoholic beverages might prove to be sufficient to evoke a conditioned aversion reaction.

As suggested earlier, historically speaking, attempts along this line on the conscious level have been made by other investigators in the so-called conditioned reflex aversion treatment of alcoholics. In these instances, the subjects were given alcoholic spirits after a nauseant and an emetic drug (generally emetine hydrochloride) had been administered. The result was that the patient would become nauseated and vomit the ingested alcohol. The purpose was to create a conditioned reflex association of nausea, based on taste and smell, to alcoholic beverages. This was repeated for a number of treatments until the therapist was satisfied that the patient had developed an aversion to alcohol. I should like to comment further on this mode of treatment. Long ago, Dercum had deprecated the use of such depressant and nauseant drugs as emetine and apomorphine in the treatment of alcoholism, considering the treatment as possibly harmful and of little lasting benefit. Certainly the treatment is not without its dangers and is, because of its duration, a painful experience for the patient. No doubt there has been some success with this method, although longer follow-up data on results obtained have been difficult to secure. The one important drawback in the treatment is that the patient is usually aware that he is being given an injection of a nauseant drug when the spirits are administered. If we are to assume that the patient associates the vomiting with taking the whiskey, why could it not just as readily be assumed that he is as likely, if not more likely, to associate the vomiting with the injection? Illustrative of this type of reaction was a 32-year old alcoholic woman whom I encountered some years ago at the Cleveland House of Correction. She had just completed a "wonder cure" at the Greenhill Institute there. It appeared that her husband had mortgaged the family car so that she could have the treatment. When I asked her why she had begun to drink again, after her husband had made such a sacrifice to have her treated, she protested, "But doctor, after they made me puke for three days and three nights, I just had to have some whiskey to settle my stomach."

With reference to the use of disulfiram (Antabuse) one must also be aware of certain problems. There are persons who may present a toxic sensitivity to the drug. Undesirable side effects such as drowsiness, mild grand mal convulsions, gastrointestinal complaints, fatigue, headache, dizziness, and diminished sexual potency have been reported. The treatment is generally contraindicated in the presence of diabetes, renal disorders, liver diseases and epilepsy. It is particularly hazardous to cardiac and hypotensive patients who drank while taking disulfiram and suffered severe reactions, as would be anticipated. In some instances such reactions could be fatal.

Antabuse can be very helpful as an adjunctive in selected cases. Posthypnotic suggestion can also be very helpful in influencing the patient to take his antabuse regularly as prescribed.

Many alcoholics will take disulfiram for a brief period and discontinue its use whenever they feel a desire to go on another drinking spree. The principal deterrent to the use of disulfiram is the fear that it engenders in the patient. Frequently, patients taking disulfiram may demonstrate a prevailing tension or manifest anxiety concerning the possible consequences, should they yield to the desire to drink.

To review briefly here, my decision to experiment with hypnosis in attempting to create an aversion was based on a number of considerations. First and foremost, I felt that one of the greatest weaknesses of the aforementioned treatment approach was that it was on a conscious level. It appeared likely that the aversion and disgust reaction could be prolonged and intensified if an associative conditioned-reflex reaction could be established in the unconscious mind of the patient and, furthermore, that in order for the aversion to persist it had to be established beyond the reach of conscious resistances and ego defenses. In addition, it was desirable to avoid the use of possibly dangerous nauseant and depressant drugs. The advisability of submitting patients who are often seriously nutritionally depleted to daily emesis for seven to ten days can frankly be questioned. It was also apparent that, if successful, the hypnotically induced reflex aversion could be established much more rapidly and effectively, without causing the patient any conscious discomfort or dread of the treatment.

It was felt, too, that the aversion reaction could be made more intense and lasting to the patient because of the greatly increased state of affectivity under hypnosis. It appears preferable for all concerned to be able to create a disgust aversion reflex reaction in a painless manner, so that the patient experiences a lack of appetite and/or lack of desire for alcoholic beverages. Obviously, such a patient will not consume alcoholic beverages if he derived no pleasure from them and actually finds that the smell, taste, and sight of alcohol upset him physically and emotionally. Finally, I found that such a treatment could be easily given on an outpatient basis and would not require the hospitalization of the person and the loss of time and expense involved.

No claims are being made for this treatment as a cure-all for alcoholism. It represents only a procedure for attempting to control drinking so that constructive psychotherapeutic, social, and economic rehabilitative steps can be taken. Alcoholism is symptomatic of deeper, underlying disturbances of the personality, and there are probably as many diverse causes for alcoholism as exist for human unhappiness and pain.

With regard to the overall procedure employed, I have found it most efficacious to give the treatment on two to three successive days depending on the patient's condition and response to treatment. Treatment should be given weekly thereafter for six months to one year in order to thoroughly condition the patient against alcohol. Psychotherapy, preferably group therapy, should be instituted immediately. After the initial treatments, patients may test themselves with alcoholic beverages. If properly conditioned under hypnosis, they will promptly become nauseated and frequently vomit any ingested spirits.

If the patient is in a poor nutritional state or in need of medical care or hospitalization, posthypnotic suggestion can be used to advantage to facilitate his cooperation in remedial measures. It is advisable to use posthypnotic suggestion further and influence the patient against the use of sedative drugs and tranquilizers as a substitute for the alcohol. The dangers of this substitute practice should be strongly stressed. Alcoholics are particularly apt to develop dependency on habit-forming sedative drugs, since they are generally suffering from marked inner anxieties, dependency needs, and guilt. As mentioned, psychotherapeutic measures should be strongly encouraged at this point and posthypnotic suggestion utilized toward securing the patient's cooperation, since the underlying personality and character problems contributing to the drinking should be dealt with.

Aside from affording the opportunity to influence the patient to pursue a constructive medical, social, and psychotherapeutic regimen by the skillful employment of posthypnotic suggestion, the hypnoreflex aversion treatment presents certain other advantages. It is completely harmless in the hands of a properly trained psychotherapist who is a qualified hypnotist. Furthermore, since it is administered under hypnosis, it is possible to keep the patient relatively consciously unaware of any painful or disagreeable nauseating or vomiting experiences. This treatment can easily be administered to ambulant patients and does not require hospitalization. Since the aversion is created at an unconscious level, it is more intense and lasting. In addition, as noted previously, it provides the opportunity, while the patient is in the hypnotic trance, to explore some of the principal problems and conflicts which may underly his alcoholism and to permit him to abreact his emotional tensions. It is often possible to better evaluate the patient's problems with regard to whether he should undergo individual or group psychotherapy or both.

The majority of patients do reveal emotional problems of varying degrees, i.e., inferiority, insecurity, sexual difficulties, depression, repressed rage, guilt, etc. Many reveal masochistic tendencies, i.e., the enraged husband who gets drunk to hurt his wife.

It is further evident that the treatment should be conducted by a psychotherapist who is well-trained in hypnosis, for hypnotherapy is a method that requires adequate comprehension of the dynamics of the unconscious mind. Much harm can be done by its misuse, and it must be used only with specific medical and psychotherapeutic indication, never indiscriminately.

Treatment is first explained to the patient as harmless, and no attempt is made to force the patient to undergo it. Cooperation should be on a completely voluntary basis.

As stated before, the hypnotic reflex aversion treatment is far more effective than conscious conditioning because the aversion is created while the subject is cortically relaxed and inhibited and cannot employ his ego defenses or resistances. There is a stronger affective component in the latter instance, because under hypnosis affectivity is markedly increased while intellectualization is markedly diminished. The disgust-aversion reaction is therefore felt by the patient with greater intensity. Furthermore, because of hypnotic amnesia, he is unable to link or correlate the aversion reaction with any administration of a drug to induce it. It appears that the conditioned-reflex treatment of LeMere *et al.* could be considerably more effective if given under hypnosis. In most instances, I simply intensify the disgust, aversion, and displeasure of the hangover state by having the hypnotized subject actually relive one of his worst hangovers.

It is important, as indicated earlier, to create, if possible, an aversion reaction to all types of spirits, including beer and wine, since I have seen instances in which a patient was given an aversion treatment to whiskey only and then attempted to switch to beer or wine in order to satisfy his craving. Again I repeat, it is most advisable to stress the dangers of switching the dependency to sedative drugs, such as barbiturates and tranquilizers, while on the other hand, stressing constructive measures.

The creation of aversion to odors can also be quite effective with such drugs as alcohol, for instance. That is, this aversion can be effective if the patient is given strong suggestions in the trance that alcohol is a dangerous poison which can penetrate the brain cells and the nervous system rapidly and cause serious cell destruction because it has lipoid soluble characteristics, that it causes extensive brain damage, brain swelling, delirium tremens, liver damage, hypertension, renal damage and marked vascular destruction. It also can cause an accumulation of very poisonous acetaldehydes and other toxic byproducts of alcohol in the blood and tissues.

I have also found that aversion reactions by means of hypnosis can be successfully induced in the treatment of such conditions as obesity (aversion to specific foods), compulsive cigarette smoking, and certain instances of narcotics addiction. This technique has proven very valuable, I found, in the dietary control of diabetic patients. If at all possible, treatment should be given in conjunction with individual or group psychotherapy, or both. Social therapy, i.e., Alcoholics Anonymous, can be very helpful, providing it does not take a stand against psychotherapy. It is wise to use the periods of abstinence to help the patient resolve underlying emotional problems.

The following cases are examples:

A 45-year old, divorced male became an alcoholic at about 20 years of age. He began drinking at the age of 16 years. His drinking followed a compulsive pattern, and after severe bouts he would become depressed. During such postalcoholic depression states he twice attempted suicide, once by hanging himself with a belt.

The patient gave a typical picture of latent repressed homosexuality; homosexual men particularly tended to disturb him greatly. He suffered from partial impotence and had strong feelings of inferiority, guilt, and self-condemnation, particularly manifest during his hangovers and brief intervals of abstinence.

He felt that alcohol relieved his tension and made him feel more masculine and less aware of the effeminate component in himself. When drinking, he would release his pent-up self-hate on others, acting hostile, becoming enraged at the slightest provocation, and being disagreeable and negativistic. He described his alcoholism as a "crutch" on which he could always lean when he felt bad: "I would just wipe out reality for about two weeks. It made it possible for me to talk more freely to others, especially to females."

My endogenic method of hypnotic relaxation was employed, bringing the patient into a medium-depth trance within five minutes. He was regressed and then made to relive his worst hangover, including the malaise, headache, nausea, and vomiting, while smelling and tasting whiskey, wine, and beer.

He was given the specific suggestion that, whenever he tasted, smelled, or even looked at alcoholic beverages, he would begin to relive these horrible hangover feelings and he would again smell the puke and vomitus. These treatments were given on three consecutive days and then repeated weekly for six–12 months. During this period he was treated by group psychotherapy weekly for nine months. This patient has been abstinent for 17 years at the time of writing. He states that he cannot anticipate any pleasure at the taste, smell, sight, or thought of alcoholic beverages.

A 56-year old woman had been a chronic alcoholic since her husband's death eight years earlier. Prior to that, she stated, she had drunk only socially and had never experienced alcoholic intoxication.

The patient stated that she frequently felt a compulsion to drink even though at times she had desired to abstain but was unable to do so. She was relaxed by the endogenic method, initially given three treatments on consecutive days and then given repeated weekly aversion conditioning treatments for six months. This patient did not have an emesis, but felt very nauseated, reliving a former severe hangover state.

She had been completely abstinent for 21 months at the time of writing. She has complete aversion to the taste and smell of alcoholic beverages. These not only evoke a disagreeable nauseous feeling rapidly but also are promptly associated by the patient with disagreeable "hangover" feelings.

A 53-year old, married man had been affiliated with Alcoholics Anonymous for eight years but was unable to curb his drinking. He had been drinking excessively for approximately 30 years. Under hypnosis he revealed that he had suffered from severe feelings of inadequacy as a man and that alcohol made him feel less anxious, more vocal and more "manly." The patient revealed further that he was a minister's son and had been reared very rigidly with regard to sex. Sexual matters were never discussed at home and the patient had always been held up as a model boy for the congregation. He was constantly plagued by shame and guilt feelings about masturbation and sexual preoccupation. After puberty he became increasingly preoccupied with perverse and infantile sexual impulses and fantasies. He always felt very guilty about these, and later in life he discovered that he could derive considerable relief of his guilt through drinking. His drinking bouts were followed by strong secondary guilt feelings, depression, and physical illness.

This patient was given an aversion treatment under hypnosis. Two days after this, while under considerable mental tension, he went into a bar and ordered 2 ozs. of vodka with orange juice. After ingesting this drink he became nauseated and had an emesis. He was given a second aversion treatment on the next day, and weekly follow-up treatments for six months. Intensive psychotherapy was instituted in order to deal with his deep-seated neurotic problems. He has remained completely abstinent for 12 years at the time of writing. His guilt and anxiety feelings have greatly diminished, while his insight into his problems is greatly improved. He has been able to remain on his job, a position of responsibility. He also reports that his marital life generally has improved.

When dealing with a married person, it is important to explore the interaction between the patient and his spouse. The following case is illustrative.

Jim was 62, a respected mechanical engineer, who had been a periodic drinker for about 30 years. He then began to drink more heavily to the point that he was frequently unable to work. It had finally reached the point where his wife of 38 years was on the point of leaving him. He recognized that he needed help although he was not too cooperative at first, acting somewhat tense and at times resentful.

Under hypnosis this patient revealed that his wife had given him an ultimatum—either undergo treatment or "I'm leaving." Jim revealed his bitterness over her being so cold and undemonstrative toward him. As a result of this disclosure, several sessions were had with his wife concurrent with weekly hypnoaversion treatments. For the first two months of treatment, Jim was on antabuse along with his hypnotherapy. He has now been completely abstinent from alcohol for over one year. His wife had been much more understanding of his needs and has, according to Jim, been very loving and encouraging. It was clear that Jim's resentment of her coldness had much to do with his drinking.

The value of psychotherapy as an adjunctive procedure to hypnoaversion with alcoholic patients is illustrated by the following case which brings out the characteristic duality generally found in the alcoholic personality.

A young, married, business executive came for treatment because of excessive drinking and marital difficulties, centering largely around his persistent infidelity to his wife, and his strange, ambivalent behavior, which was incomprehensible to the wife.

Following a hypnotherapeutic session in which aspects of his relationship to his parents were explored, this patient had the following highly interesting dream. He was on a hillside in his native mountains, looking into a clearing, when he saw a beautiful fawn. He became fascinated with the beauty of the animal and tried to lure the fawn to him. A doe was following the fawn. Suddenly, on the other side of the clearing, a hunter appeared with a long rifle. The patient was immediately disturbed by the thought that the hunter was intending to shoot the doe and cried out, "You wouldn't shoot that doe in front of its fawn, would you?" The hunter angrily replied, "Wouldn't I? Just watch me." The hunter then took aim and shot the doe between the eyes. The patient cried bitterly, "Now you've gone and done it," and awakened sobbing. In his discussion of the dream the patient points out that for a fleeting moment it seemed like the hunter was himself and then the image seemed to merge into the identity of his father. "Father," he said "was like that . . . brutal, heartless, many times sadistic. I recall," he said, "how terribly upset I felt when father abused mother in front of us kids." The patient recognized that at times he could be cruel and heartless like his father. It was this part of himself that made him feel guilty and which he detested in himself. But, on the other hand, he pointed out, "Sometimes I am warm and protective like I was toward the fawn in the dream. That's the way mother is." In further discussion the patient recognized that this maternal, submissive component was what appealed to his present wife, since she was the dominant person and took the initiative in love. On the other hand, he pursued numerous extramarital affairs, pursuing rather naive, innocent, submissive girls, whom he repeatedly hurt. This pattern he recognized as similar to his father's. It is clear that his Oedipal conflicts were still unresolved and psychotherapy obviously indicated; the patient made excellent progress.

HYPNOAVERSION IN THE TREATMENT OF OBESITY

In 1959, I reported on my new treatment procedure for the treatment of oral compulsions, such as alcoholism, by means of hypnotic aversion. Because this technique proved valuable in controlling compulsive drinking, as noted earlier, I later employed this procedure in the treatment of nicotinism and initially reported on that work in November 1965. This treatment proved to be quite effective. It was possible to improve the technique so that positive results, in patients sincerely desiring to stop smoking, were over 75 percent after one to two years follow-ups. Encouraged by these results, and in view of the fact that most individuals who give up cigarettes begin to gain weight, I sought to test this hypnoaversion procedure in the treatment of compulsive overeating.

In the treatment of eating disorders hypnosis was induced by my endogenic technique first presented in 1957. While under hypnosis the patients were given suggestions that they would regress and relive a past nauseant and highly disagreeable earlier experience of a toxic type, i.e., alcoholic hangover, food poisoning, intestinal flu, nausea of pregnancy, etc., while tasting or ingesting bread, fats, oils or sweets. Part of a piece of toast with margarine, sugar or artificial sweetener was introduced into their mouths with the suggestion that they would feel revolted and nauseated by the poisonous, ugly, fat-producing foods, the starchy bread, the greasy oily fats, the sickening sweets, etc. A little low grade cooking oil helps to make the experience even more disagreeable. These suggestions were coupled with suggestions that they would feel sick, nauseated and poisoned just as they felt when they had the unpleasant past toxic experience. It should be noted that a past nauseant, disagreeable experience can be readily reexperienced under hypnosis as though the patient were experiencing the original disgusting episode (hypnotic "revivification"). To facilitate the recall and create the association of a disagreeable "hangover," for instance, the specific alcoholic beverage on the palm or on a sponge is held under the nose of the patient, while the subject is tasting the so-called "ugly, fat-producing" foods. The terms "sickening hangover" and "ugly, fat-producing" are repeated to establish the association in the subject's mind. Further, the association of "poisonous" and "nauseous" helps the patient to relate the effects to his previously experienced toxic nauseant episode. It is highly effective to correlate a past nausea and vomiting of pregnancy with the "sickening, revolting, ugly, fat-producing foods."

The success of hypnoaversion depends a great deal on the patient. Some patients have difficulty in recalling past traumatic nauseant experiences. Since in the hypnotic state recollection is heightened, it is often possible to help patients to more easily recall a past nauseant experience while under hypnosis. If the past experience is sufficiently traumatically nauseant, it is easier for the patient to develop an associated reaction with the specific toxin or harmful foods.

The patient is commanded to put a hand on the sensitive area where he once felt the worst nausea. When attempting to create aversions to specific foods, one should have the patient extend the tongue and then place toasted bread with margarine and sugar (or artificial sweetener) on the tip of the tongue, offering the suggestion that it will taste disgusting, nauseating; then move it to the middle of the tongue suggesting it is now going to be much more sickening, revolting and nauseating. Next the food sample is placed on the back of the tongue and pushed gently toward the throat suggesting that the subject will begin to feel very nauseous and feel like vomiting. Toast is best because it can be introduced more easily and deeply into the patient's mouth and creates a strong nauseant reaction. It is suggested to the patient that he will first experience dry heaves which will get progressively worse and intolerable. He is instructed that he should tell the therapist when he can no longer tolerate the food in his mouth. At this point the nauseating food is removed and the tongue cleansed. It is then suggested that he will not become ill again unless he eats starchy, greasy, or sickeningly sweet foods and that as long as he adheres to the proper diet of fresh fruits, vegetables, lean meat, nonfried sea food and other healthful, low caloric foods that are on his dietary list, he will not become nauseous again and will feel fine.

While hypnotized, patients were given the suggestion that the low caloric foods, i.e., salads, fruits, and fat-free proteins, in their special diets would taste better than ever. It is good to suggest citrous fruits, melons, nonfried sea food, lean meats, etc. Further, they are given strong instructions that they limit their total caloric intake of the low calorie foods or they will feel uncomfortable.

The patient is then told that he will be given an "antinauseant compound to inhale (i.e., a placebo consisting of a pleasant aromatic). The patient is given the suggestion that after inhaling this "delightful, antinauseant, antispasmodic," he will feel warm, relaxed, and comfortable all over—in his stomach, his throat, and all through his body. At this point additional, positive instructions, for example, for healthful exercise, recreation, can be given, following which the session can be terminated. The patient is awakened by the standard counting-out procedure.

In the first reported series of weight cases where this hypnoaversion procedure was employed, 50 patients were treated. Forty-nine were successfully hypnotized. Weight loss varied from two to 11 pounds per week. Average weight loss was four pounds per week. All of the patients who were hypnotized lost weight. Those who were initially more obese usually lost weight more rapidly. As the patients were conditioned by repeated treatments, weight loss was usually greater due to the rigorous regime of diet and exercise and the progressive potentiation of the hypnotic effect. One patient discontinued treatment after previous marital difficulties came to a head.

Over many years of practice since those initial studies, I have found that the treatment of markedly obese persons by this method has proven surprisingly effective. Some illustrative case examples follow.

Mary was 31, mother of two children, recently separated, severely depressed and suicidal. When Mary had tried medication, Weight Watchers, reducing salons, dieting, it was all to no avail. When she had reached a weight of 320 pounds, her husband left her. There were no doubt other reasons. Mary had a poor self-image that seemed to extend beyond her weight problem. Because of obesity, Mary would hardly appear in public. She was extremely self-conscious and self-deprecating. She was a sedentary personality who had never participated in athletics, hardly ever danced and except for her household duties, did virtually little. She was obviously so desperate that her cooperation in treatment was obtained without difficulty.

Under hypnoaversion treatment in which she would reexperience the nausea and emesis which she had had during early pregnancy every time she tried to eat starchy, fatty or sweet foods. She was made to delight in salads, citrous fruits, lean meats and other dietary low-caloric foods while avoiding fried sea food. Under hypnosis, she was also instructed not to partake of even low-caloried foods in excess of the prescribed dietary regime. She was given the suggestion that if she felt any hunger between meals or in the evening, she would eat citrous fruit or have a salad. Post hypnotic suggestions were given that she would begin to enjoy physical activity and recreation, i.e., tennis, swimming, bicycling. In a relatively short time she took up tennis and soon after bicycling. She was receiving weekly treatments.

At first her weight loss was marked, from seven to ten pounds weekly. Later, it dropped off gradually. She lost a total of 190 pounds in one year, averaging slightly less than four pounds per week during that period. She has grown quite attractive and has become an active, joyous person. After one year, she weighed 137 pounds and was able, as a result, to obtain an excellent job.

Of interest is the fact that during treatment when Mary weighed 160 pounds she would still not appear in public very much. As she put it, "I can't understand it. I have lost so much weight and I still feel fat." It was my impression that Mary's self-image had not yet changed. She was suffering from a sort of phantom obesity. As she continued to lose weight and gained increased insight, the phantom obesity dissipated.

It is now over one year since treatment was completed on Mary. She currently weighs 145 pounds and has not regained. Her eating and living habits have become radically changed and she is optimistic and hopeful about the future.

In another case, a 46-year old woman weighed 365 pounds and complained of feeling depressed and unhappy in her marital life. Since she had gained so much weight, her husband's sexual interest in her had markedly declined. In addition, she was suffering from hypertension and experienced some dyspnea on moderate exertion. She admitted she had been very self-condemning, felt insecure and disturbed at her husband's loss of interest. She stated that she loved him very much and desired to correct the situation. Apparently she had been so emotionally upset that she was now frigid at times.

Hypnoaversion therapy was instituted with prompt results. She lost 12 pounds the first week. She has lost 80 pounds in the first three months of treatment. She has been quite active playing tennis, swimming, etc. which was stimulated by posthypnotic suggestion. She was given the suggestion that as she lost weight, she would feel greater sensuality and sexual response. After one month she reported greater sexual desire and response. She noted increased vaginal secretion. After the second treatment, she reported that her sexual activity had increased to the point that she had coitus with her husband three times in one day and experienced multiple orgasms. There is a remarkable change for the better in her behavior, mood, and zest for living.

The advantages of employing hypnotic conditioning are apparent. As explained earlier, the patient is not only conditioned against high-caloric foods, but is influenced hypnotically to enjoy dietary low-caloric foods more than ever. In addition, patients who tend to gain weight usually are habitually sedentary. I have employed hypnotic suggestion very successfully in motivating them to a much more active life involving both work and recreation, i.e., tennis, golf, swimming, dancing, walking, exercising, cycling, etc. In this way the patient is not left in a void, but with a positive program of healthful diet and exercise. The patient is conditioned to a way of life that is both healthful, physically and mentally. Patients have invariably commented that the treatment was pleasant and they they experienced no conscious discomfort. They felt that they had lost a desire for the high-calorie foods; and they no longer had to struggle with cravings for such foods. As they became more active and lost weight, their moods changed from despondency, depression and inertia, to elation, feeling active and energetic. They were usually more outgoing and along with an improved self-image began to relate better to others.

There is the further advantage of not becoming habituated and dependent on drugs, often not without harmful side effects, in order to control weight. Invariably, once they stop taking such drugs, they regain the lost weight. With my procedure the patients become so thoroughly conditioned to proper diet and exercise that they rarely ever regained weight after treatment was terminated. The great majority of obese patients have emotional problems underlying their compulsive eating. Some develop secondary problems as a result of their obesity, i.e., inferiority, depression, self-hate, social anxiety, etc.

A further advantage of this procedure is that while the patient is under hypnosis, causative problems can be explored so that an attempt can be made to resolve them. Some of the common underlying causes of overeating are:

1. Eating as oral substitute for love (emotional starvation). For example, as in the case of a 22-year old, comforting himself by gorging himself with food whenever he felt rejected by a female

2. Eating to relieve tension

3. Eating for defiance and spite: masochistic type (Resentful of nagging, i.e., to spite parent or husband, etc.)

4. Eating compulsion (anxiety). I had the occasion to hypnotize a young, obese woman of about 30 who prior to the induction asked if there were any way to determine the cause of her eating compulsion. She was regressed to the age of four, whereupon she recalled a scene in which the mother cat was feeding the newborn kittens and she asked her mother, "What will happen to the kittens if the mother cat dies?" The mother responded, "If the mother cat dies, then the kittens will die." Since then, she had seemed to always link eating with maintaining health and life and

warding off death. After this was consciously ventilated, her eating compulsion began to disappear. The excessive compulsive eating no longer made sense. As a matter of fact she came to recognize that the overeating was much more of a deterrent to good health than a benefit.

5. Eating because of boredom, loneliness, and depression

6. Eating because of pathological craving, i.e., diabetes, etc.

7. Eating to avoid sex (Fat becomes an armor and defense against inadequacy).

Of interest is the case of Linda, 22-years old, who had come in for hypnoaversion weight-reduction treatment. After two sessions following which she had begun to lose weight, she became somewhat anxious and decided that she desired to interrupt the weight-reduction treatment. Under hypnosis she revealed that she had had four abortions and in two there were complications which could have been serious.

As a result of these traumas, she had virtually interrupted her sexual activity. Under hypnosis, she explained further that on one occasion the male had literally raped her, on another had threatened to kill her if she didn't submit. She began to feel safer when she felt overweight, less attractive and had lost much of her sex appeal.

It is important to recognize the problem of the patient who desires hypnotherapy for obesity and has the basic attitude of wanting someone to overpower her in a magical fashion and make her do something she doesn't really want to do. This is an erroneous assumption. One should not attempt by means of hypnosis to make a patient do something she doesn't desire to do. Rather, hypnosis can most effectively be employed as an adjunct to assist a person in achieving diet-control, proper exercise, and if possible, the elimination of disturbing and painful tensions. The latter two factors cannot be ignored and should be resolved, if at all possible. Patients who are depressed or overanxious may show poor motivation as regards treatment. Hypnosis can provide an excellent means for rapidly getting at the root of such tensions and correcting them if the patient so desires. That is, through the use of hypnotherapy, underlying conflicts can be explored and eventually resolved.

This treatment could undoubtedly prove very effective in controlling the dietary and exercise habits of cardiac, hypertensive, diabetic, hypoglycemic patients. It has proven valuable in controlling excess weight during pregnancy.

Where the obesity was associated with more serious emotional conflicts, psychotherapy was employed both on an individual and group level in an attempt to resolve these. While the patient was under hypnosis, it was possible usually to quickly uncover the cause of these conflicts and other aggravating factors. Due to the positive, supportive treatment regime, no notable emotional side effects were observed.

When patients employ oral, regressive or fixated behavior to allay tensions, to pacify or comfort themselves, it is best to provide oral substitutes, i.e., for the alcoholic the suggestion of the use of fruit juice, fruit, soft drinks or candy. This has the added advantage that sugar reduces the craving for alcohol. For the cigarette smoker, substitutes may be suggested depending on individual preference, gum, mints, cinnamon sticks, etc. For the excessive eater, suggestions are given that low-calorie foods will taste wonderful. It is explained to the patient that such foods can provide sufficient compensation for the deprivation of high-calorie foods.

This is a completely safe procedure which can achieve long-term favorable results because of a resulting persisting, radical change in dietary, exercise and overall living habits. Such conditioning in regards to diet, exercise and living habits, occurs more rapidly and effectively with the aid of hypnotic influence.

HYPNOAVERSION TREATMENT OF NICOTINISM

Due to recent investigations with reference to the role which tobacco plays in the etiology of such conditions as bronchiogenic and throat cancer, hypertension, angina pectoris, peptic ulcer and other conditions, considerable numbers of patients have requested the aid of hypnotherapy in breaking a severe smoking habit. Toward this end, the author has employed hypnosis in creating an aversion to cigarettes and tobacco products.

Many of the nicotinists I have treated have suffered from chronic organic conditions, such as emphysema, chronic bronchitis, myocarditis, coronary and vascular disease, hypertension, peptic and duodenal ulcer. A considerable number of these cases were referred for treatment by their physicians. Approximately 90 per cent suffered from symptoms such as dyspnea on moderate exertion (climbing 15 to 20 steps), persistent smoker's cough, throat irritation, dryness in mouth, laryngitis, gastritis, excessive expectoration, anorexia, weight loss, insomnia, poor peripheral circulation with cool extremities and increased fatigability.

The rationale of the hypnoaversion treatment of smokers was to establish a strong aversion-conditioned reflex response to tobacco by means of hypnosis. Since the patient is hyperaffective and obsessional in the hypnotic trance, it is possible by means of hypnotic suggestion to fixate strong aversions beyond conscious awareness. It is further possible to create a greater antipathy against existing side effects which aggravate the patient and intensify the desire to rid themselves of such symptoms, i.e., a persistent cough or bad taste in the mouth, etc. (I use the term "smoker's halitosis.") It is further possible to regress patients to organic and physiological reactions associated with smoking, bronchitis, laryngitis, dyspnea and to emphasize the great value of abstinence in preventing these conditions.

The patients were treated without previous hypnosis-susceptibility tests or interviews in order to determine the percentage of successful inductions and response to treatment, which would be achieved with unselected subjects, individually or using group treatment. An average of three treatments were given within the first 72 hours, during which the patients are likely to experience maximum withdrawal discomfort. In my first reported series, one hundred cases were treated individually. Another hundred in groups of three to five at a time.

Of the first hundred patients inducted individually only 11 failed to go into a trance on the first induction. Of these, three were successfully hypnotized and treated on the second visit. Of the one hundred who were treated by the group method, 84 were successfully hypnotized on the first attempt. Of the remaining 14, only three could be hypnotized on the second attempt, and this was done privately. As a result of improved technique, I now have satisfactory inductions of 96 per cent.

My endogenic respiratory method of induction was used, plus standard trance-deepening procedures, such as hand levitation, reverse counting, and circumduction. The average induction time was five minutes. This did not vary much in the two groups, except that in most cases the group induction appeared slightly more rapid. Average number of treatments given were six, three on successive days as mentioned, and then staggered.

In the previous studies on alcoholism and homosexuality, it had been found that markedly unpleasant taste and smell sensations could be induced by suggestion in the hypnotic state. These are actually induced regressive perceptions which are related to earlier association. The following aversion procedure was employed. In half the subjects treated, an attempt was made in the hypnotic trance to induce a strong aversion to the taste and smell of cigarette tobacco alone. Suggestion was employed to induce a nauseous reaction, spreading from the throat to the lips, upon contact of the tobacco with the throat, tongue or lips. This taste aversion was augmented by a suggested nauseant reaction resulting from smelling the tobacco. Taste and smell aversion was potentiated by regressing the patients to experiences of nausea or vomiting following the ingestion of poisonous drugs, alcohol or foods. The suggestion was given, "You will become nauseated and sick, just as you did that time you ate the poisonous meat, etc." The patient then usually relives the sickening effect.

In some cases, particularly those averse to lung irritation with fears of asphyxiation and disturbed by dry, persistent coughing, the patient was instructed to inhale deeply and to hold his breath (until he experienced a strong urge to cough.) In addition, it was suggested that the patient will experience the fumes in his lungs as highly irritating, poisonous, disagreeable and nauseating. The nausea reaction is potentiated by the previously experienced oral-alimentary nausea.

The latter procedure provided the additional advantage of creating an aversion reaction to the filter tipped cigarette. It was suggested to the patient that he would feel and react to the poisonous fumes coming through the filter tip with coughing and a sense of choking.

As stated, an attempt is made to regress the patient to the most nauseating, disagreeable gastrointestinal upsets the patient had experienced preferably from food, alcohol, or as a result of intestinal flu toxemia, nausea of pregnancy, or postoperatively.

I found the great majority of patients are able to consciously recall an earlier, disgusting, nauseating experience without difficulty prior to induction. Sometimes, however, the recall of such an experience is facilitated by questioning in the hypnotic trance. Illustrative of this was the following case of a 46-year old nurse who had been smoking for about 25 years and had been smoking between two and three packs a day. She was suffering from Raynaud's disease and her hands and toes were frequently cyanotic and cool to the touch. Although she could consciously not recall a nauseant experience, under hypnosis she recalled that she had become nauseated following an injection of sodium pentothal prior to surgery. She was then given the hypnoaversion treatment. An injection of pentothal was simulated while a cigarette was placed in her mouth. It was strongly suggested that everytime she tasted or inhaled a cigarette, she would reexperience a similar, sickening nausea to that which followed the pentothal injection.

During the treatment, she developed a nauseant reaction to the cigarette and was given posthypnotic suggestion that everytime a cigarette was put in her mouth or inhaled, she would relive the same nausea and that this would be intolerable to her. Some hours after treatment she told a friend, another nurse, that she was sceptical about the effectiveness of the treatment and stated that she was going to test it by trying to smoke a cigarette. She then did so and over a period of about ten hours smoked approximately one third of a pack. She told her friend, "You see, it hasn't even affected me. The treatment didn't work." After ten hours passed, however, she became extremely nauseated. She attributed this to some food she had just eaten at dinner and also believed it might be due to a small amount of champagne she had drunk. She tried to light another cigarette to settle her stomach but became still more nauseated. She stated that at that point she realized what had happened. She had told me she had become nauseated right after the injection of the pentothal, but actually she recalled that she had become nauseated after coming out of the anaesthetic postsurgically.

Interestingly, this patient never felt a desire to smoke subsequent to the experience, but nevertheless received two follow-up treatments. She has now been abstinent from cigarettes for five years and her Raynaud's condition has disappeared completely.

This case illustrates that the individual experiences the past nauseant traumatic experience in exactly the same time sequence and association as it actually happened—a point that is of key importance in terms of the treatment procedure in hypnoaversion therapy.

Occasionally a patient is encountered who cannot recall ever having had nausea or vomiting. It is best to then ascertain what has been the most distressing, disagreeable feelings that he had ever experienced from smoking, drinking, or overeating, etc. Some will recall discomfort and pain, headache, palpitation of the heart, precordial pressure, dizziness, coughing, spasms, choking sensations, faintness and general weakness, etc. Sometimes the patient is able to recall more distressing symptoms under hypnosis that can be utilized to advantage. These upsetting symptoms can then be correlated with the smoking, drinking, overeating, or other destructive habits, i.e., nailbiting, scratching, etc. While the patient is in the trance, it is best to explore emotional factors, i.e., in smoking, the matter of allaying anxiety, in drinking, seeking escape from feelings of failure, working off rage, reliving tension or inferiority feelings, etc., in overeating, attempting to relieve boredom, loneliness, frustration, anxiety, disappointment, etc., feelings of rejection, lack of affection, pent-up resentment, etc.

Under hypnosis, recollections of revolting, disgusting, nauseant episodes are facilitated. In some instances, the patient cannot recall such experiences that have left a traumatic impression. If, for example, the patient dreads the effect of cigarettes on his heart or lungs, the following approach is often quite effective.

After the patient is hypnotized, a cigarette is placed between his lips and he is told that he will receive a poisonous injection of nicotine through the cigarette because that is the way he draws that poison into his body when smoking. If he is concerned about his heart, suggestions are given that nicotine is weakening the heart and that the pulse will have to be controlled so that the patient will not receive a dangerous amount of poison. Suggestions are given that the pulse is becoming rapid and weakening. Then suggestions that the heart is beginning to miss beats, indicating that the nicotine is causing a serious circulatory deficiency in the coronary and heart circulation. Then suggestions that the pulse is beginning to disappear. The hypnotist exclaims his concern over this reaction and at this point, the cigarette is removed and the patient is told to rapidly exhale the poisonous nicotine. Then he is given a fragrant stimulant to inhale (placebo) and told that this contains an excellent coronary dilator, heart stimulant, and will rapidly restore his heart function to normal. The hypnotist expresses relief that the patient recovered from the toxic reaction.

If the patient is concerned with his lungs, he usually dreads asphyxia. The cigarette is placed in his mouth. If possible, cigarette smoke is blown strongly into his nostrils. He is given the suggestion that he will experience a very unpleasant asphyxiating (choking and burning) sensation in the throat and lungs. He is told that the choking sensation gets progressively worse as the poisoning continues and will soon become unbearable.

When he feels too uncomfortable, the cigarette is removed and he is told to breathe out the poison rapidly and he will receive the inhalant, a powerful bronchodilator and antispasmodic and that his breathing passages will promptly open up. (This is in reality merely a fragrant placebo solution, as mentioned earlier.) He is warned that under no circumstances will he ever again put a cigarette in his mouth as this could rapidly produce a choking seizure again.

Of interest was the case of a 51-year old male patient suffering from marked emphysema and hypertension as a result of heavy smoking (100 cigarettes daily). It was found that he had a strong aversion to the smell of burnt rubber. He was hypnotized and regressed back to the burning rubber trauma while the cigarette was placed between his lips. It was suggested that it would taste like burnt rubber. For several treatments a rubber band was burnt near his nose while suggestion was given. Actually, he stopped smoking completely after the first treatment. Additional treatments were given to reinforce the aversion. He has been completely abstinent from cigarettes for over nine years.

An effective procedure to enhance the awareness of the damaging effects of tobacco is the following which can be done after the hypnoaversion procedure.

The patient under hypnosis (preferably in a medium or deep trance state) is instructed to exhale. It is suggested that his body is getting smaller and smaller—tinier and tinier—so tiny that you'll be able to enter your own body and see the damage that is being done to you by the poisonous tobacco. It is suggested that a microlite will be inserted first to illuminate the throat, then the larynx, then the trachea and bronchi. The patient is then instructed to visualize the damage done by the tobacco. Usually he will make the observation that the throat is reddened and irritated, that the voice box is irritated, reddened with brown splotches and that the trachea and bronchial mucous membranes are covered with black (tar) and brown (resins) areas. It is suggested that these are dangerous carcinogenic accumulations which will disappear after the patient stops smoking. After the patient has seen enough organic damage to be impressed, the microlite (usually a large fountain pen), is removed. The patient is then told to breathe deep to reexpand back to his normal size.

In summary, under hypnosis, the patient's defensiveness and sensitivity to dangerous noxious substances can be increased. Specific intense anxiety can be thus stimulated and then rapidly alleviated by suggestion plus the appropriate aforementioned measures. We have learned from observation of neurotic, compulsive patients that obsessive avoidance reactions are common. Compulsive avoidance behavior always has anxiety at its roots.

Patients can be beneficially reassured and positively motivated by telling them as they are recovering from the toxic effects of the cigarette, etc. under hypnosis that they demonstrate an excellent heart recovery rate and will enjoy wonderful health once they are totally free of the poisonous cigarette.

When the treatment is given, the patient must always be told that he will only become ill if the poisonous cigarette is in his mouth or inhaled into his lungs directly but that anyone smoking around him will not affect him in any way.

I should like to report on a typical case, that of a 45-year old married woman who had been smoking one and a half packs daily. She had been smoking for approximately 25 years. She presented in treatment because of concern about a persistent cough and shortness of breath when climbing steps. She was advised by her physician that she had no cardiac abnormality and that the dyspnea was due to her excessive smoking. She was warned by him that she showed early signs of emphysema.

The patient was easily hypnotized. Strong posthypnotic suggestions were given that the patient must immediately give up smoking due to the dangers which it presented for her health. Existing symptoms, such as the cough and shortness of breath, and the danger of developing emphysema, were utilized as strong deterrent factors. In addition, she was made to feel that these were the fore-

runners and warning signs of much more serious consequences to her health, such as the likely possibility through
increased susceptibility in middle age to such conditions as
angina pectoris, coronary occlusion and bronchiogenic carcinoma, and that she must heed these warnings.

This patient presented some resistance in that she expressed her fondness for the smell and taste of tobacco.
This was countered under hypnosis by having her smell
and taste an old burnt-out cigarette, which obviously had
a very disagreeable odor. It was then strongly suggested to
her that after smoking as she did, her breath smelled like
this old burnt-out cigarette and was very unpleasant to her
husband and others. Furthermore, while still under hypnosis the patient was instructed that the residue tars, resin and
ash that she tasted were the cellular irritants that over a
longer period of time could produce smoker's bronchitis,
and throat and lung cancer. This procedure seemed to
make a deep impression on the patient and when, soon
after awakening, she was offered a cigarette, she shuddered
and turned away from it.

This patient had one follow-up treatment two days
later in which the initial suggestions were reinforced under
hypnosis. She has now been abstinent for approximately
four years and has not the slightest desire for cigarettes.

Certain patients can be hypnotized better individually.
On the whole, however, it is possible to attain good results
with group treatment if at least one highly susceptible,
sensitive and cooperative patient is present in each group.
The strong aversion response of this patient, who of course
should be treated first, greatly heightens the aversion reactions of the others in the group. Such interaction is analo-
gous to the nausea experienced by passengers on a ship
tending to create nausea in other passengers—a kind of
"contaminating suggestive mechanism" or "sympathetic
response."

It was noted in general that results can be greatly improved by close follow-up treatment, particularly in the initial stages.

It was found that underlying factors contributory to nervous tension and the patient's tension-release dependency on cigarettes could be uncovered and, in some instances, satisfactorily resolved. In some cases, by means of hypnotic suggestion, it was possible to substitute harmless methods of relieving tension, i.e., chewing gum, candy, cinnamon sticks, etc. Posthypnotic suggestion was given in instances to encourage physical and mental recreation. Under hypnosis it was possible also for people to ventilate pent-up tensions and concerns. The catharsis thus achieved usually helps a patient in combating his smoking.

It is best to reinforce treatments for greatest effectiveness. After an initial three consecutive daily treatments, another treatment should be given one week later, then two weeks later, and then at monthly intervals for approximately six months. After that, at three to six month intervals for one year, or, as indicated, by the patient's response to treatment.

Spacing treatment sessions in this manner also facilitates follow-up on the progress of patients.

It must be kept in mind that hypnotic suggestion should be utilized to assist patients in accomplishing the desired objective, in this instance, giving up smoking. It is generally unwise to give such treatment to patients who do not really desire to stop smoking, but are relying on hypnotic suggestion to force them to give up a crutch which they are really unwilling to relinquish. In some cases it is best to attempt to resolve resistance or to postpone treatment.

There are those who have argued against the hypnotherapy of smokers on the grounds that if the patient gives up cigarettes, he will probably develop serious reactions or substitute symptoms. I have not found this to be the case in the patients I have treated. In general, there has been not only an improvement in physical health on abstinence, but also a lessening of anxiety and nervous tension. I recall a patient, a newspaperman, who was being kidded by his colleagues to the effect that "We understand that if you give up smoking, you will develop something worse," whereupon the patient smiled and remarked, "Well, if you mean that in treating me, the doctor also cured me of my impotence—yes."

Certainly the assumption is fallacious and negative that a destructive syndrome or reaction must necessarily follow the removal of an unhealthy, damaging symptom or habit. Why couldn't a positive, healthful habit be induced instead?

A prime objective which the treatment achieved was to lessen or totally eliminate the appetite for tobacco. This removed the continual painful wrangle over whether or not to light up just one cigarette—a constant struggle for the smoking addict.

The treatment was always considerably more effective if the smell and taste of the cigarette could be correlated by hypnotic suggestion with specific symptoms, symptoms that the patient has already noted. It is well to stress that continued smoking usually causes such specific injury to one's health and eventually leads to the development of conditions such as coronary disease (smoker's angina), cancer, emphysema, hypertension, etc.

Heavy stress should be placed on the important benefits of tobacco abstinence in terms of good health and longevity and of freeing one's mind of the continuous burden of anxiety which smoking causes in such patients.

Generally, it was noted that patients unconsciously struggled harder toward positive goals of good health than they did to avoid the harmful effects of cigarettes. Some even maintained an unconscious attitude of defiance concerning smoking as if they were fighting a demanding, critical authority who was trying to deny them their desired pleasure. Such attitudes need to be discussed. The patient must realize that the doctor will only help him to do what he, the patient, wishes to achieve.

Often the patient's overall "will to live" was a decisive factor in his responding to treatment or in seeking treatment. Some patients who failed in treatment after initial success revealed unconscious, self-destructive tendencies or a rather feeble "will to live." They were usually at cross purposes with themselves.

Encouragement for a joyous, full and active life appeared an important factor. In some cases, excessive anxieties and insecurities concerning the job, marriage, etc. contributed to relapse to smoking. Another prime cause of relapse to smoking was excessive drinking. Alcohol is a cortical depressant and decorticating agent and tends to temporarily block the hypnotic and posthypnotic conditioning. If the patients tend to drink excessively, they should be given hypnoaversion treatment against alcohol prior to the tobacco aversion.

The particular problems of the individual patient should be evaluated in treatment and, whenever possible, dealt with to reduce anxiety and the compelling need for an addictive crutch.

OTHER CONSIDERATIONS IN THE APPLICATION OF HYPNOAVERSION THERAPY

Hypnoaversion therapy opens a new field for clinical research. Aside from its use in obesity, nicotinism, alcoholism, it opens up the possibility of being helpful in the treatment of drug addiction in general. Hypnoaversion has also proven useful, I have found, in the treatment of nail biting. In addition, it could be of benefit in chronic lip biters, skin pickers, nose pickers, etc.

Most patients presenting themselves for hypnotherapy have never been hypnotized. Consequently, they may be anxious, sometimes outright fearful of being hypnotized. Some are curious and some are quite sceptical. Many are markedly ambivalent. They may desire to for example give up smoking, drinking or excessive eating for health reasons but then add, "But I enjoy smoking, etc." Intellectually they have decided to try to give up the harmful habit, but emotionally they are in conflict between their anxiety and the gratification they experience from smoking, drinking or overeating. The prime aim of the hypnoaversion therapy is to make these harmful practices revolting and unpleasant. This eliminates, for the most part, the ambivalent conflict that goes on in the minds of many such persons.

Anxiety as regards treatment is usually best relieved by exposing the patient to other patients who have responded well to treatment. They not only alleviate the new patient's anxiety, but because of their favorable attitude toward the therapists and the benefits of therapy can help to improve rapport and suggestibility. An attitude of trust greatly facilitates successful treatment. The importance of this factor is illustrated by the following case example.

A woman was given the hypnoaversion treatment for obesity. She responded so well in the first session that she promptly vomited during the session when sweets were put in her mouth. She had been a compulsive candy eater. She recovered from her nausea and went out into the waiting room. Inadvertently, the nurse asked her how her stomach felt now after being so sick. This question was asked in the presence of two new patients. As a result both of these patients became quite anxious. The next patient had to be reassured because she expressed anxiety about becoming sick. She then entered the treatment room and although somewhat refractory I was able to treat her. However, because of her apprehension, she entered into a light hypnotic trance. However, she emerged in the waiting room feeling fine and as a result the anxieties of the third patient were lessened. Nevertheless, the third patient also showed some degree of resistance, but was still able to respond satisfactorily to treatment.

Thus, it is clear that negative reactions manifested by other patients can greatly affect treatment. Examples of patients responding well, on the other hand, can be very helpful and may spell the difference between success and failure. In some instances, curiosity and anxiety can be allayed by having the new patient observe the hypnotic induction of a responsive patient.

If resistance is encountered initially, it should be dealt with promptly. The underlying causes should be probed. Patience and a kindly, understanding attitude are very important. In many instances resistance can be successfully resolved. The patient is often grateful to have been helped to overcome his anxiety and to accomplish the desired result.

Resistance is manifested under many pretexts, for example, being ill and unable to come to treatment or having to take care of something that is very important. Some resistance is manifested early by attempts to resist hypnotic induction or to simulate induction. Highly interesting was the reaction of several women who, as they were reaching a deeper level of hypnosis, cried out, "No, no, no," which can happen in women who have a resistance to giving up control and experiencing an orgasm in coitus. This is in contrast to the type of patient who, when she is approaching the deep hypnotic level, confronts it with serenity and an attitude of feminine surrender and is more apt to feel in a, "Yes, yes, yes" mood. Some defiance takes the form of trying to smoke in spite of the disgusting, sickening, nauseating effects. There are some patients who are quite masochistic and will smoke in spite of the fact that it makes them very ill. Some of these patients reveal a good deal of subconscious guilt, defiance or self-directed rage.

It is best to be certain that the patient is in a sufficiently deep trance before administering aversion treatment. If the patient carries out hand levitation and the extremities are limp, the muscles hypotonic, he is ready for the treatment. If the patient goes into a light trance, it is usually better to give suggestions that he will go much deeper the next time. He can then be brought out of the trance and either be reinducted immediately or on the next day. Each time he goes under, it is suggested he will go deeper and the treatment will become increasingly effective. This fact should be repeatedly suggested during each session.

Patients who have been defiant toward parental and adult authority as children may still manifest this defiance by attempting to maintain control and resist induction and treatment. Such conflicts must be ventilated consciously.

In general, I have found results were more favorable in those patients motivated to take the treatment because they had a serious organic condition, i.e., as pulmonary emphysema, early coronary disease, chronic bronchitis, asthma, Berger's disease, peptic ulcer, hypertension, etc. These patients were prepared earlier for hypnotherapy by their physicians who pointed out how seriously smoking affected their medical condition. There are many cases where the use of drugs to counteract smoking or religious-educational approaches or warnings on cigarette packages did not appear to be very effective in helping patients to stop smoking. On the other hand, persons who were pushed into treatment by members of their family, etc. might often consciously or subconsciously sabotage the treatment as if to prove that they shouldn't have been pushed in the first place. It is good to keep in mind that "push" often creates "counterpush." It often evokes earlier childhood resistance reactions.

In brief then, to review some important procedural points to assure the maximum effectiveness of hypnoaversion treatment with new patients: If the patient has been prepared for hypnotherapy by another patient who had gone through the treatment successfully and is very eager and positive in his attitude, his chances for successful response to treatment are greatly enhanced. If the patient reveals any skepticism or doubt, tends to be uneasy, restless, or preoccupied, it is best to discuss such matters and to defer treatment until the patient is in a more susceptible frame of mind. If the patient reveals any trace of anxiety, it is far better to discuss such anxieties, before making any attempt at hypnosis. Those patients who exhibit fears of loss of control and insomnia often are difficult to hypnotize. In such cases, it is far better to have one or two preliminary sessions before any attempt is made. It is also very important that the hypnotist explain that he is first going to run a preliminary test, that the test will be very pleasant, and the patient can feel very free to relax. During this preliminary test, above all, the patient's suggestibility and capacity to concentrate must be observed carefully. If the patient passes the susceptibility test (see pp. 00 and 00), it is suggested he is ready for deeper induction and will more likely comply with further suggestions, thereby attaining a deeper level of hypnosis. In short, the patient is hypnotized during the test thus reducing defenses and circumventing defenses. This has an important advantage. If the induction fails, it is the patient who has not passed the test and not the hypnotist who has failed. Since the prestige of the hypnotist is not hurt, he is in a better position to work through resistances and make subsequent induction attempts.

GROUP HYPNOAVERSION THERAPY

When group hypnoaversion treatment is employed for smoking, alcoholism, or obesity, it is helpful to keep the following points in mind:

After the group is hypnotized, it is best to give the suggestions of the reliving of the sickening nausea to one of the patients who has already experienced a marked nauseant reaction under hypnosis to the cigarettes or alcohol. The nauseant reaction of this initial patient triggers off a marked dread of nausea and lowers the threshold of the rest of the group to reexperiencing the sickening nausea reaction as though it were a kind of chain reaction. This care in selecting one or even better two patients who have been very responsive to the treatment can greatly improve the prospects for successful treatment. I have found that nauseant-disgust reactions could be markedly potentiated by playing a tape of the reaction of a patient who suffered intense nausea and vomiting accompanied by loud sound effects. Such a recording can precipitate marked nauseous reactions.

As I have indicated earlier, it is most helpful in the preparation of new patients for hypnotherapy and in particular, hypnoaversion therapy, to expose them to successful patients in the waiting room—as though it were accidental. A receptionist can casually introduce the patients to each other using their common interest in combating smoking or seeking weight loss as a starting point of conversation. There is virtually nothing that has so strong a positive suggestive value as the presenting the *fait accompli* of the therapeutic success. The old adage that "Nothing succeeds like success" certainly applies in hypnoaversion treatment.

REVIEW AND FURTHER EVALUATION OF HYPNOAVERSION TREATMENT IN ALCOHOLISM, NICOTINISM AND WEIGHT CONTROL

It is about twenty years since I first applied my hypnoaversion procedure which I have since improved and modified somewhat. However, the basic approach has remained the same except for modifications in techniques. The results have been increasingly gratifying.

More recently, I felt that I had now ample clinical data to review and better evaluate the results and technique with the objective of improving the procedure.

As noted earlier, patients were hypnotized by my endogenic procedure and given strong suggestions that they would reexperience a previous nauseant episode of a toxic type (i.e., alcoholic hangover, food poisoning, intestinal flu, nausea of pregnancy, etc.) while smelling or tasting alcoholic beverages, cigarettes (in nicotinism), or specific high-caloric foods (in obesity).

Under hypnosis, there is a marked loss of discriminating ability and a high degree of intellectual abstraction coupled with hyperaffectivity. Hence, the taste or smell of a toxic cigarette for instance can be correlated with the toxic nausea occurring in gastrointestinal flu.

The patient under hypnotic regression can only relive what he had originally experienced. Therefore, suggestions should be given that the same precise past, nauseous reactions (e.g., vomiting) will reoccur every time the patient smells or ingests the harmful substance. That is, appropriate, specific suggestions are repeated that the patient will feel sick, nauseated and poisoned precisely as he/she had felt when the patient had the disagreeable past toxic nausea.

Thus, when applying this procedure in the treatment of alcoholism, for instance, after being conditioned, every time the drinker smells the alcoholic beverage or attempts to drink, he can be induced to automatically relive his worst hangover experience. It has as a result been possible to cause alcoholics to become averse and disinterested in alcoholic beverages, for alcoholics rarely ever desire alcohol during the hangover phase. Similar aversions can be made to a number of harmful substances, in particular tobacco and to certain addictive drugs, i.e., heroin, morphine, etc.

In terms of the frequency and duration, hypnoaversion treatment for alcoholism was administered weekly for four to six months depending on the patient's progress, then biweekly, and then monthly.

As for adjunctive procedures, I have found that hypnoaversion treatment has been highly effective in the treatment of alcoholism in conjunction with Antabuse at the onset and supplemented by group psychotherapy and social therapy. While under hypnosis, the etiological psychosocial pathology underlying the drinking should be explored.

In nicotinism cases, treatment with few exceptions was limited to six treatments given as aforementioned. However, in more resistive cases, the number of treatment sessions was increased. Some merely reduced the number of cigarettes smoked at first and clung at times desperately to their oral pacifier. In such cases, it was necessary not only to step up treatment, but also to suggest acceptable substitute pacifiers, i.e., cinnamon sticks, hard candy, their favorite gum as well as encouraging recreational and social activity. Much oral escape in our culture appears to be due to boredom, inactivity and depression as well as to tensions, anxiety, resentment, guilt, etc. Treatment for smoking was administered daily for three days and then staggered one week later, then two weeks, a month and then as required.

Many smokers associate cigarettes with alcoholic beverages or coffee—in much the same way that bacon is associated with eggs. It is good to break up this pleasurable association by suggesting that the alcoholic nausea experienced will enhance the cigarette nausea. Likewise, the nausea experienced in tasting and smelling tobacco will make coffee taste bad and that vice versa coffee will increase the nauseous reaction to tobacco. Thus, what formerly in-

creased pleasure now increases the aversion reaction—
breaking up the habitual association of pleasure.

Whenever possible, as indicated earlier, it is best to
take the patient back, using regression and high degree of
suggestibility so that he will relive an earlier toxic experience, such as the worst alcoholic hangover, and to correlate
this experience of being poisoned, the nausea, dry heaves,
gagging, and sometimes vomiting, directly with the smell
or taste of a cigarette which is placed close to the nostril or
on the tip of the tongue. This nauseant association can be
enhanced by letting the patient smell liquor at the same
time. The slightest smell of a cigarette will then be associated with the nauseant experience. In some instances,
patients are unable to recall such a poisoning experience,
but recall their first encounter with cigarettes, which caused
choking and dizziness. It is then possible by lighting a cigarette, blowing the fumes in his face, placing it under the
patient's nose or in his mouth to cause him to relive the
same reactions. This procedure is often effective where
other methods might fail.

It is of great importance to explore the side effects
which smoking causes patients, i.e., cough, excessive mucous secretion. Shortness of breath and hyperacidity and
the other symptoms which the patient has experienced and
has had concern about generally form an excellent basis for
convincing him while he is in a trance that the cough and
the irritation of the bronchial cells are a warning sign of the
body, and that continual irritation of the bronchial cells can
cause malignant degeneration to cancer and other damage,
i.e., emphysema, chronic bronchitis, bronchiectasis, and
lower resistance to tubercular infection. It is best to dwell
on the organ of primary concern, if it is the heart, then on
possible heart damage. If it is hypertension, then the effects
on blood pressure, pulse, coronary, shortness of breath
(dyspnea), fatigability. If the primary concern is the lungs
or gastrointestinal tract, then it is best to use possible seri-

ous injury to those areas as deterrents. Furthermore, the shortness of breath which the patient has personally experienced, he is told in the trance, is an indication that the circulation is under severe embarrassment and stress and that all the arteries of the system are constricted, including the coronary artery, and that it is no wonder that one is short of breath. The patient must act to prevent any serious trouble. Clinical experience has shown that patients with some organic disease are not hard to convince that they must stop smoking. The patient, under a trance, is more suggestible, and his fear defenses can be greatly intensified so that he can be put into a much stronger mood in terms of warding off something which is dangerous to him. Since the fear of the impending danger of disease is heightened, it is strongly impressed on the patient, that the giving up of smoking would totally relieve him from a nightmare of fear of cancer, emphysema, smoker's angina pectoris, heart failure, hypertension and other horrible conditions. He can look forward to future good health as he acts wisely and realistically in totally renouncing smoking. Immediate gains should be mentioned, i.e., that the cough will stop, the blood pressure and pulse will become normal, that he will no longer tire easily or be short of breath, that his mouth will lose the bad odor and smell clean and fresh.

As for the optimum number of treatments given, I believe that after the initial course of treatment which, in the treatment of nicotinism involves three visits on three consecutive days, it is best to reinforce the treatment after one week and if necessary, as often as possible until a very strong aversion reaction is established. It is best to be flexible in one's approach to treatment, and if a patient does not show a strong aversion reaction after three or four treatments, it is best to explore the reasons why he has not responded. Sometimes the original earlier truama was not impressive enough, more often the patient is resisting going into a deep enough trance. For those patients who simulate a trance, it is best to test their responses, i.e., posthypnotic suggestions, such as counting from one to ten and omitting one of the numbers or carrying out a task after coming out of the trance. The follow-up treatments are generally of short duration and can become increasingly effective as time goes on. As indicated earlier, there are patients who show no outright aversion to cigarettes even after four or five or six treatments, but later develop a very strong aversion which can be lasting. The determining factor more often seems to be the decision of the patient as to whether he really wants to give up smoking, and that giving up smoking is a very important step for him. In other words, he is not engaging in a game to see if the doctor can overpower his will and make him do something that he really doesn't feel like doing. Many patients enter treatment as the result of an intellectual decision, even though they really do not feel like giving up smoking. They enjoy smoking too much and they are too dependent on cigarettes. Such patients rarely do well in treatment.

An interesting prognostic indicator is giving the posthypnotic suggestion that the patient leave his cigarettes on the secretary's desk (if he has any with him) before he exits. I have found that when the treatment is effective patients will leave their cigarettes. Not leaving their cigarettes is a poor prognostic sign.

In a follow-up study of 1000 smokers treated by the hypnoaversion method, after one month 90 percent were found abstaining; after three months, 82 percent; after one year, 68 percent. In a recent follow-up of 150 patients treated for alcoholism 92 percent were found abstaining after one month; after three months, 79 percent; and after one year, 62 percent. All heavy drinkers and particularly those who showed a chronic long-term drinking pattern were given 0.5 gm. Antabuse daily until the aversion was well established. Of 100 patients treated for weight control problems, 91 percent achieved weight loss after one month; 94 percent after three months; and 93 percent after one year. Of the latter group, after one year 59 percent of the total patients treated achieved "marked" weight loss and 34 percent "partial" weight loss. ("Partial" weight loss is defined here as a loss within a range not exceeding 50 percent of the patient's desired weight loss; "marked" weight loss is indicated by a loss of 50–100 percent of the desired weight loss.)

If patients are smokers to begin with, those who give up alcohol or drugs may often increase their smoking. Likewise, it is generally true that patients who give up smoking tend to eat more and pick up weight. This is due not only to the fact that nicotine reduces persistalsis and appetite but because of the need of such patients for an oral pacifier and comforter. Excessive eating or drinking after giving up cigarettes represents compensating oral needs. It is therefore best to initially suggest oral substitutes, cinnamon or licorice sticks, gum, fruit, celery, carrots and other harmless substitutes, depending on which the patient might prefer. It is further true that many patients are accustomed to have a cigarette with their coffee or cocktail. It is best to discourage the latter practice at least until the cigarette abstinence is well established.

With regard to the relationship between alcohol and hypnoaversion treatment, not infrequently patients who drink excessively relapse to smoking. This is due primarily to the fact that the effects of hypnotic conditioning are cortical. Alcohol acts as a decorticating agent thus temporarily knocking out the conditioned inhibition and aversion. As indicated earlier, extending follow-up treatments over a longer period is very advisable.

The tobacco aversion treatment has proven understandably of particular benefit to patients with cardiovascular disorders, emphysema, gastroduodenal ulcers, chronic bronchitis, laryngitis, etc. In the treatment of nicotinism, a word of caution should be noted. It is important to give posthypnotic suggestions that the patient will experience an aversion reaction only if a cigarette is put into his mouth or inhaled and *not* if he is exposed to others who are smoking.

Hypnoaversion therapy aimed at diet and weight control has proven very beneficial, often when other procedures failed. The rationale is not only to create a strong aversion to high-calorie foods, but to help the patient better tolerate and derive more pleasure from low-calorie diets. It is clear that such an effective method of diet control can be of significant value in diabetes, hypertension and cardiovascular disease, obesity, in pregnancy and other conditions.

It is to be noted that while the patient is under hypnosis, he should be strongly influenced to engage in enjoyable forms of exercise, tennis, swimming, cycling, rowing, dancing, etc. This is particularly important in that many overweight individuals have sedentary tendencies. Furthermore, those doing more mental than physical work frequently tend toward overweight conditions and obesity.

Treatment for obesity was usually administered once weekly for periods varying from three to 18 months depending on the patient's response and extent of the weight problem. In exceptionally refractory cases, treatment was given two or three times daily. Not infrequently when there are accompanying emotional and marital problems at the basis of the overeating, these need to be dealt with and, if possible, resolved.

I recall an instance in which an attractive young, married woman consulted me for her overweight condition. I pointed out that not infrequently married women who tend toward excessive weight have passive, undemonstrative husbands. She promptly responded with, "That's the problem in our marriage, but it's no use, my husband would never go to a psychiatrist." I asked if her husband cared about money. "Does he," she exclaimed, "he's so security conscious. I was afraid to tell him I had consulted you for fear he'd gripe about the money it cost."

"How do you suppose he'd react," I asked, "if you were to tell him that I could teach him how to give you the follow-up hypnoaversion treatment and he could as a result save quite a lot of money." "I think that would work" was her answer.

Her husband, a rather passive, physical scientist came in a bit apprehensive at first to be sure. He gave a very limp handshake. To make a long story short, he was instructed in giving the treatments to his wife. The results were remarkable. His wife became quite attractive and slender in the ensuing months and he became a much more secure, demonstrative and assertive husband which pleased his wife greatly.

In considering hypnoaversion treatment, the following factors are of importance:

1. The selection of patients
2. The training and skill of the hypnotherapist
3. The ability to deal with resistance
4. The degree of cooperation and insight of the patient
5. The cooperation of the spouse or parents
6. The susceptibility of the patient to hypnotherapy
7. The frequency and duration of treatment
8. Participation of the patient in individual and/or group therapy to attempt the resolution of emotional causative factors
9. The availability of adequate follow-up treatment. More follow-up treatments over a longer period can only improve the results and careful attention should be given to need for continued follow-up treatment.

The prognosis in hypnoaversion treatment is excellent if the patient desires to cooperate in giving up drinking, smoking, overeating, etc. Too often patients are pushed into treatment by their spouse, parents, boss, etc. It is important to stress that for best results the patient should be in agreement with the treatment objectives. An intellectual decision to give up these indulgences does not have the necessary emotional motivational force behind it. Too frequently, it is based on a rationalization that perhaps the hypnotist can make me do something I really do not wish to do. In such instances, the individual often regresses to the adolescent, defiant state unconsciously and struggles against the forbidding parent, namely, the hypnotist. Thus, the patient seeks to defeat the treatment to counter the authority he had always resented. This attitude is best dealt with by the therapist through clarifying his role as merely desiring to help the patient accomplish what he desires, and by explaining that the way to achieve this is by mutual cooperation. Most patients can and do develop strong aversions to alcoholic beverages, cigarettes and certain foods even though they were initially resistive.

The effects of posthypnotic suggestion and conditioning vary greatly. Sometimes the effect of treatment wears off rapidly. To insure the best results it is useful when possible to give follow-up treatments monthly or bimonthly for some time until the conditioned response is firmly established and the patient has sufficiently resolved his emotional problems so that alcohol, nicotine, food and drug props are no longer necessary. There is no harm in continuing follow-up treatment for several years. The question of length of treatment required is best left to the therapist's judgement.

In my opinion, the results of the hypnoaversion treatment can be significantly improved by the following steps:

(1) Psychotherapy.

Due to the fact that alcoholics and obese patients usually have emotional problems underlying their excessive and compulsive drinking and eating, psychotherapy is necessary. For example, frequently women married to rather undemonstrative husbands tend to "comfort" themselves by overeating. Such patients benefit from the postive love "strokes," emotional support and recognition that they receive in group therapy. This is to a large part responsible for benefits that obese women have obtained with the "Weight Watchers" and other reducing groups. I have found that women may overeat when they feel resentful toward their husbands for neglecting them, showing little affection or failing to appreciate their efforts and contributions. Conflict, apprehension and boredom are responsible for much excessive eating, drinking and smoking. Attempts are made to resolve these difficulties often by bringing the husbands into group therapy so that they can better comprehend the needs of their wives and vice-versa.

Again, I should like to emphasize that those who have addictive-compulsive tendencies to overeating, oversmoking and drinking are generally in need of psychotherapeutic assistance. Individual and, in particular, group therapy are advisable. In groups these individuals gain emotional support and reinforcement against their compulsively destructive tendencies by the examples and encouragement of others. The group therapy also helps such individuals to resolve emotional conflicts in their interpersonal relationships and to further maturity. Most oral neurotics cannot be regarded as fully emotionally mature.

(2) Suggestions for exercise are given to the patient. (That is, to increase physical, recreational and work activities and the benefits stressed.)

(3) Intensive follow-up treatment of the patient. (Patients usually respond positively to a continued interest in their condition by the therapist.)

Of interest is the fact that all of these excessive eating,

drinking and smoking activities contribute to the development of hypertension and heart disease.

It is to be noted that hypnoaversion treatment does not cause the patient any conscious distress or discomfort. Patients generally describe the treatment as agreeable. It has the great advantage of rarely requiring hospitalization.

HYPNOTIC-AVERSION TREATMENT OF HOMOSEXUALITY

For many years there has existed a widespread tendency to disparage the use of hypnosis in the treatment of homosexuality. Clinical experience has amply demonstrated that psychoanalytic treatment of homosexuality is relatively ineffective and prolonged.

Arguments presented to deprecate the use of hypnosis in the treatment of homosexuality have been that hypnosis: (1) tends to make male homosexuals more passive; (2) tends to further infantile regression and dependency; (3) tends to further homosexual attachments between hypnotist and patient; and (4) tends to lessen the patient's feelings of responsibility.

As Meares stated the position, "The passive male homosexual enjoys the hypnotic trance and obtains erotic satisfaction in the intensity of hypnotic rapport with the therapist." Such a patient, in Meares' opinion, may report improvement in his homosexual condition in order to mislead the therapist into continuing the hypnotherapy which affords him erotic satisfaction.

Stekel wrote that, "The proper psychotherapeutic method can never be hypnosis. What may we expect hypnosis to accomplish as long as the homosexual has not learned to acknowledge openly the response against which he had fought so long? Contrary to Krafft-Ebing, Schrenknotzing and Alfred Fuchs, I have never met with a lasting cure through hypnotic treatment." Stekel declared that, "regardless of the type of treatment, we must accept only with the greatest caution the statements of homosexuals who claim to have been cured by us." In my opinion, the acknowledgement and recognition of his neurosis is not sufficient. The homosexual patient must desire treatment. By means of hypnoaversion therapy he comes to feel resentment, disgust and aversion to invert practices and to consciously reject homosexuality, as well as to develop positive heterosexual feelings and desires. It follows that those homosexuals and in particular, bisexuals, who are in conflict with and somewhat disturbed by their homosexuality have a better treatment prognosis.

My rationale has been based on Freud's pleasure principle and the efforts of the unconscious mind to relive a pleasurable and to evade or avoid a painful, disgusting or disagreeable experience. Pavlov had demonstrated how conditioned reflexes can be established and how reactivity can be so intensified that a slight stimulus can produce a marked and complex response. It is known that the phenomenon of hypnosis resembles a conditioned response in that the subject becomes increasingly susceptible to hypnotic induction. It is similarly possible to "sensitize," intensify and accelerate a conditioned response by means of hypnosis. In the case of alcoholism and nicotinism, I developed procedures whereby the odor or taste of an alcoholic beverage or of cigarette tobacco would be sufficient to trigger a marked aversion reaction. It was found possible to condition patients under hypnosis to such an aversion to these substances that even the mere thought of the word "alcohol" or "tobacco" could elicit feelings of revulsion. I have found that attempts to condition alcoholics by means of emetic drugs is not nearly as effective or rapid as is the conditioning of alcoholics by means of suggestion in the hypnotic state.

My decision to experiment with hypnosis in attempting to create aversion reactions was based on a number of considerations. First and foremost, I felt that one of the greatest weaknesses of treatment in the nonhypnotized state is that resistance to suggestion and conditioning is often overwhelming. It appeared likely that the aversion and disgust reaction could be prolonged and intensified if a conditioned reflex reaction could be established in the subconscious mind of the patient and, furthermore, that in order for this aversion to occur and be fixated, it must be established beyond the reach of conscious resistances and ego defenses. Furthermore, the conditioned association and aversion reaction can be more prolonged because of posthypnotic amnesia.

I found that the aversion response could also be made more intense and lasting to the patient because of the greatly increased state of suggestibility, concentration, affectivity and reactivity of the individual in the hypnotic state. It seemed preferable to be able to create a conditioned aversion reaction so that the patient not only experiences immediate revulsion on physical contact with a homosexual but also comes to anticipate such contact with feelings of disgust, displeasure and dread. It appeared also that if an aversion can be accomplished by hypnotic suggestion that an attraction to the opposite sex could be likewise established. Research needs to be attempted without preconception or bias. I desired to objectively evaluate the value of hypnotherapy in the treatment of male homosexuality and bisexuality.

Clinical experience has revealed that those who turn to homosexuality have been preconditioned by a faulty rearing process which has caused them to reject their natural sexual roles and practices. In general, it seemed that there might be a possibility that those functional conditions which are a product of such faulty emotional conditioning of the child by parents, teachers, etc. might be corrected, in certain instances, by a suitable emotionally corrective reconditioning therapy. Where the faulty conditioning incorporates certain specific aspects of sensory aversion and pleasure it may be possible to alter such reactions and induce natural healthy responses instead. In short, by means of hypnotic suggestion and conditioning, I have been able not only to create deep aversions in the male homosexual to the male body, but on the other hand to reduce or relieve disgust, anxiety and horror reactions which such patients may have toward the female body and female genitals. It has, in fact, been possible to make the female body very attractive to such individuals.

This procedure with which I began preliminary investigation in 1959, has thus far been attempted on 13 male patients ranging in age from 26 to 40. The first patient reported in this series began treatment 17 years ago, and the endogenic induction procedure was used throughout. In selection of these patients such factors as suggestibility, desire for and acceptance of treatment and insight were considered. In general, it was found that male homosexuals are quite susceptible to hypnotic induction. Eleven of the 13 patients reported can be termed bisexuals, in that they periodically manifested some conscious and unconscious heterosexual desires. One patient had never revealed any sexual interest in females prior to treatment. Only three had ever consummated a natural heterosexual act, whereas all had indulged in perversion, six of them, admittedly, with females.

In general, I found many male homosexuals, and in particular the effeminate, passive type, possess a rather high degree of sensitivity to specific sensations of smell, taste and touch. Like females, they are particularly sensitive to body odors and use deodorants and perfumes extensively. Further, they tend to be fastidious, sometimes compulsively clean, and are often averse to a lack of cleanliness and personal hygiene on the part of their sexual partners. A majority of the male patients selected had already experienced specific traumatic disgust reactions with certain male partners. Under hypnosis I found it was possible to exploit such sensitivities and aversions by regressing these individuals back to the time of their most disturbing disgust reactions. Then by means of this revivification it was possible to potentiate those reactions and those past feelings, causing these patients to either affectively relive such unpleasant reactions or to induce and establish marked revulsion reactions while in the trance. Posthypnotic suggestion was also given to the effect that these same "disgust reactions" would recur whenever they were in intimate contact with a male body. After a number of conditioning sessions under hypnosis, these patients became highly sensitive to close contact with homosexual males, perceiving them as foul smelling, filthy, disgusting and distinctly unpleasant. The most revolting odors were found to those of urine, feces, stale perspiration and bad breath. One of the cases seen very recently by me revealed considerable revulsion to the odor and taste of semen and tended to associate it with the odor of Chlorox. Suggestions of filth associated with the male genitalia and anal areas of their partners were implanted in their subconscious and reinforced periodically during the hypnotic trance. It was further suggested to the patients that because they were particular about their own personal hygience, they were especially revolted by the uncleanliness of other males. This was to prevent any excessive sensitivity or disturbance about their own cleanliness.

Since the aversion reactions created under hypnosis were so prompt and effective, several sessions were usually sufficient to establish a strong aversion reaction to males. Periodic reinforcement treatments were given during the first year at monthly intervals. At the same time, reinforcement of attraction to females, particularly a specific one in whom the patient is or could be interested, is given, and contact with the opposite sex was strongly encouraged by means of posthypnotic suggestion.

Thus, I have in similar manner repeatedly utilized hypnotic suggestions to establish deep-seated aversion in many individuals to alcohol, tobacco, certain addictive drugs and specific foods. Further, such aversions could be established much more rapidly and to far greater intensity than could be accomplished, if at all, in the nonhypnotized state. The basic consideration here is that early homosexual erotic experiences are associated with pleasure and that the homosexual desires to relive these early pleasures. Furthermore, the homosexual has usually come to associate pain and rejection with the opposite sex and pleasure and acceptance with his own. Thus, if the pleasurable associations can be converted or diverted to disgust reactions, and these responses sufficiently established by hypnotic suggestion, the individual might conceivably be repulsed rather than attracted.

By means of hypnotic regression and revivification techniques it is sometimes possible to take the subject back to his earliest homosexual experiences and to elicit specific disagreeable impressions which can then be markedly potentiated by hypnotic and posthypnotic suggestion.

It is clear that the homosexual neurosis is complex and the total personality of the individual is involved to varying degrees. The homosexual neurosis is sometimes active, sometimes latent and repressed. Faulty sex identification and aversions to the fulfillment of normal sexual roles are manifest. Deep-seated fears of castration frequently need to be resolved. Typically there is a lack of attraction to the opposite sex.

Psychotherapy of such conditions involves the establishment of emotional corrective transferences leading to healthy sex-role identification, and the resolution of pathological defenses and reaction formations.

I had occasion to treat a young man, 25 years of age, who had recently been married. Soon after the wedding, B. took off, leaving his newly acquired bride, in, to say the least, a state of consternation. He had taken her life's savings—several thousand dollars, and gone to his boyfriend in Florida where he rapidly dissipated the money. He then contacted his parents and told them he needed more money very badly. The parents were very distressed over the whole matter. It was a small town and everybody soon learned of his shameful, outrageous conduct. The parents told him that they would only help if he consented to accepting treatment. So B. came to me. His initial attitude was that it was all one big joke. He promptly told me that if his boyfriend called him, he wouldn't be able to resist and would probably take right off for Florida.

I hypnotized him without too much difficulty. He was treated on successive days during which he was conditioned to an increasingly stronger aversion to the male body and at the same time conditioned to an increasing attraction to his wife's body. Fortunately, his wife J., was most helpful and followed my instructions carefully, acting warm, accepting and encouraging. One day after he had been in treatment for about three weeks, J. came in and complained that B. had been acting harshly, self-centered and inconsiderate toward her. At that point, I had already established a good rapport with B. and he was rather surprised when I turned on him sharply and castigated him rather severely. In fact, he was so disturbed, he almost terminated treatment at that point. I had previously instructed J. to act sweet, kind and accepting in spite of his having been disagreeable. This maneuver worked beautifully. From then on B. showed marked progress toward a healthy heterosexuality. He made what appears to be a complete recovery in two months of treatment. It is now 12 years since his treatment and he and J. are getting along splendidly with each other and their three children.

The rationale of having B. become disillusioned and resentful towards the therapist and getting warm acceptance and understanding from his wife tended to disrupt his positive feelings towards males and greatly strengthened positive feelings towards his wife. Apparently, B. was extremely upset and traumatized when I was severe with him. A strong affective reaction of this kind often can precipitate a marked change in terms of the choice of a love object. His effort to gain my acceptance and compromise my authority at this point was apparent. The potentiating effect of hypnosis on transference-affective reactions is often remarkable.

Reconditioning therapy based on the pleasure-pain principle is highly important since the pleasure principle is so strongly operative in such states. By exploiting the pleasure-pain (disgust) responses, it is therefore possible to induce marked aversion to the male body while enhancing attraction toward the female body as a whole. Posthypnotic suggestions that homosexual males have a putrid odor are enhanced by the patient inhaling a putrid odor during the fantasied confrontation with a homosexual. On the other hand in this treatment the patient is given the opportunity to fondle soft cushions (simulating the female breasts) and inhale a most delightful fragrance. (It is important to see that the female partner involved uses a similar fragrance.) The patient can likewise be made to experience an aversion to the hard bony muscular body of a male which he comes to associate with the putrid odor. Hard objects wrapped in cloth (simulating the hard, bony, male body) can be pressed against the patient.

My procedure is not to be mistakenly regarded as a cure-all. It is in its experimental stage, and though promising, cannot be considered even at best as more than an adjunctive procedure in the treatment of this complicated condition.

There is every indication that similar results can be attained with female homosexuals. Thus far I have had only one case, and this patient has done splendidly. She is now enjoying a gratifying, normal heterosexual relationship and strongly desires marriage and children.

These procedures should in any case be accompanied by longer term individual or group psychotherapy.

Hypnoanalysis was employed by the author to facilitate the recollection of early traumatic and significant emotional experiences. I feel that by means of hypnoanalysis additional insights may be gained in understanding prime causal factors of the patient's homosexulaity and furthermore what is needed to counteract the inverted desires.

Hypnotic suggestion should be used to influence the patient to a greater degree of independence, assertiveness and initiative in his normal role. It is further used to encourage the process of separation from inverted and destructive personality components and the acquiring of positive appropriate and healthful characteristics.

All of the cases herein reported were given psychotherapy in conjunction with hypnotherapy. The following cases are illustrative:

The first case was that of a student seminarian, aged 26, who was expelled from college for homosexual acts. This patient was markedly effeminate in his feelings, speech and mannerisms. He demonstrated strong mother identification. Under hypnosis it was learned that during one of his early homosexual encounters with a noncircumcized male he had experienced a revulsion to the smell and taste of urine and stale perspiration. He was also revolted by the smell of excretions and sweat. It was possible by potentiating and intensifying the revulsion under hypnosis to create a marked aversion-nausea-disgust reaction toward the male body as a whole, with resulting strong disgust reactions in the area of smell as well as taste. After the first treatment under hypnosis his favorite lover visited him from out-of-town, crawled into bed with him, whereupon the patient promptly left the bed, feeling nauseated and uncomfortable and immediately broke off the relationship. This reaction was completely unanticipated by the patient himself, who evinced marked surprise. Only a week earlier, prior to the hypnotherapy, he had expressed strong homosexual longings for this person. Soon afterwards he broke off all contact with homosexuals. This treatment was accompanied by a number of sessions in which, under hypnosis, certain feminine attributes of females which he found desirable were potentiated and his attraction in general to women markedly increased. This patient soon began actively dating women and has felt particularly attracted toward two quite feminine girls of his acquaintance. Formerly, if he dated girls at all they were of a rather masculine type, undemonstrative, reserved, with small breasts and hips. This type is no longer attractive to him. Although he formerly had pleasurable homosexual dreams, his dreams became full of conflict, in that he was both attracted and repulsed; the attraction component of the dreams has lessened, while tendencies toward withdrawal and disgust with males in the fantasies are more marked. His smell and taste aversion to males began to occur in his dream fantasies persistently. Hypnotherapy was employed in conjunction with both individual and group psychotherapy.

A most interesting case was the following that occurred seventeen years ago. A high school teacher, aged 38, was referred by a psychotherapist who treated him unsuccessfully for several years. He was a bisexual who had been virtually impotent with his wife during the ten years of their marriage. Whenever she actively expressed a desire for sex, he felt threatened, angry and withdrew. He was somewhat effeminate in manner and speech and revealed strong maternal identification although he expressed respect and a fondness for her, he complained of a lack of sexual interest in his wife. Under hypnosis he revealed that his first erotic experience involving physical contact with a male had been with his father as a child of five. His father had been sixty when the patient was born, and was recalled only as a quiet, passive, weakly old man. "He would be pleased when I got into bed with him and lay close to him. I don't remember mother and dad sleeping together."

He remembered the unpleasant, sweaty odor of his father and further elicited regarding his hard, bony body, mostly skin and bones. It was possible to regress him back and create a strong association of a foul, disagreeable, sweaty odor of his father's body. Strong suggestions were given specifically to establish strong associations of unpleasant odors and physical revulsion regarding the male genitalia. In addition, suggestions were given associating the hard, bony body of his father and males in general as distinctly unpleasant. The patient was also revolted by the odor of feces and urine. This was reinforced by correlating the suggestion of foul, sweaty odors with those of fecal and urinary excretions and associating these with the male body. The patient rapidly developed a strong sensory aversion to males and rapidly broke off all contact with homosexuals. On the other hand, he was made to visualize and feel his wife's body as beautiful, soft, fragrant and desirable. He was conditioned to enjoy a certain perfume fragrance which his wife was instructed to use. He soon began to manifest normal potency.

Initially, as this patient became able to attain and maintain satisfactory erections and engage in coitus, he had some difficulty in ejaculating. Hypnotic suggestion aided his ejaculating. He would usually complain of pain in the urethral and bladder areas of a constrictive, spasmodic nature, during or immediately following ejaculation. This was found definitely related to marked castration fears. Under hypnosis he revealed that he felt rage and tension whenever his wife made him feel that she was demanding his attention and sexual love, and he felt obligated to gratify her. This he felt keenly to be an unjust demand upon him. He resented most of all being pushed. He felt, as he put it,

"She is using me," and considered it inappropriate for her to expect him to take the initiative and make aggressive love to her. Having lived with a passive husband without gratification for so long, it is understandable that she would have become active and aggressively demonstrative toward him. It was found that when she followed the therapist's instructions to act passive and seductive, to act almost indifferent, to withdraw and thus make it necessary for him to take the initiative completely, the patient no longer experienced pain and discomfort, felt considerably less rage and anxiety and showed a lessening of neurotic feelings and increased masculinity and aggressiveness. It was obvious that he felt quite threatened by her demands on him to be sexual and masculine. This increased his castration fears. Because of his strongly inverted effeminate feelings, he had felt angered by her demands for sexual love. His neurotic component desired to be passive and loved by an aggressive male lover. He has in the course of treatment undergone a complete change. He is now the father of a fine son, the husband of a happy, gratified wife, and is himself a happy and fulfilled man.

A follow-up study of this patient one year after treatment was begun revealed that he was participating in an active and increasingly gratifying sex life with his wife, averaging three to four coital experiences weekly. Throughout, he was highly potent.

Another illustrative case was that of a graduate student, aged 32, who had never consummated a heterosexual experience, and also exhibited marked sensitivity to perspiration and fecal odors. This patient had a strong feminine identification and exaggerated sensitivity to cleanliness and neatness. He was meticulous about his dress in spite of his meager finances. He had a platonic relationship with a female graduate student with whom he felt much in common in terms of overall life interests and goals. Although they were close friends he had never approached her sexually. He satisfied himself periodically by male homosexual experiences or homosexual masturbation fantasies. He was given the hypnoaversion treatment daily and rapidly developed a strong revulsion for male contact. The physical attractiveness of his girlfriend was strongly potentiated by means of suggestion. Three weeks after treatment was initiated he had his first coital experience and was gratified at the pleasure they both experienced. Since then, for the past year, they have been having gratifying sexual relations regularly and are planning to be married soon.

An additional case of interest is that of a night club entertainer, aged 29, with a history of active homosexuality since puberty. He related that he had never felt any sexual desire for females although he frequently associated with attractive female entertainers in the course of his career. This patient was found to be sensitive to the odors of stale sweat, urine and feces. Hypnotic suggestion was employed to potentiate these disgust and nauseous feelings and to strongly associate them with odors of the male body. On the other hand, he was given strong suggestions regarding the attractive fragrance and loveliness of the female body. Following the initial treatment, he promptly broke off all homosexual activity, complaining of increased tension, headaches and insomnia. For a brief period Valium, 10 mg. t.i.d. and Doriden, 0.5 gm. were given for relaxation and rest. His tension was fairly well-controlled with the above medication.

For several weeks this same patient complained of a marked loss of sexual feeling. He began to have dreams of burly men pursuing him and trying to hurt him. This was interpreted as evidence of his repressing homosexual desires and a manifestation of his castration fears. After two months of treatment, the patient expressed a slight amount of sexual interest in a woman of forty whom he had known for many years and with whom he felt relatively secure and comfortable. Positive suggestions then were given under hypnosis to increase his sexual desire for her and to encourage this desire to active expression. He soon reached the point where he enjoyed petting with her and for the first time caressed a female breast. He then reported a fantasy of having normal sexual relations with her. After six months of treatment he had gratifying sex with her and younger females and manifests no further homosexual interest for the last six years and is pursuing a normal heterosexual life.

TREATMENT OF HOMOSEXUALITY: EVALUATION OF RESULTS

Reconditioning a male homosexual's physical reactions to other males obviously does not alter his basic attraction to needs for love from men nor his anxieties about and hostility toward women. Physical aversion to men, however, makes possible a withdrawal from the seeking of homosexual sexual gratification and enhances the likelihood that the patient may attempt to make sexual contact with females, especially if attraction to the latter is enhanced by hypnotic suggestion. It also facilitates a desexualization of the feelings that he has towards the males he cares for.

In the case of the 38-year old bisexual for example, it was possible to bring about insight and offer encouragement to his wife so that she would be appropriately responsive when he took the initiative. The aim here is to make the posthypnotically induced experience as pleasurable as possible. This is most significant in that it is necessary to counteract the homosexual's dread and anticipation of displeasure in regard to heterosexuality.

This treatment has the best possibilities of success with bisexuals. If the male patient has an attachment to a female, such positive feelings can be intensified while disgust and aversion feelings are generated toward males. It is clear that to turn the sexual feeling off toward his own sex and leave him in a void is not conducive to a positive therapeutic result. Sexual feelings sooner or later must find a gratifying outlet.

This treatment does not offer a too favorable prognosis for the strongly fixated homosexual in whom a sexual interest towards females is neither manifest nor can be aroused.

Since these aversion reactions set up in the homosexual are of a cortical type, they tend to be blocked by alcohol or drugs which depress cortical functions. Alcohol, of course, further tends to release cortically repressed homosexual desires, as was noted in a case cited previously.

In my studies of the application of hypnosis in the treatment of homosexuality, I have attempted to evaluate the comparative effects of posthypnotic suggestion and hypnotic transference on therapeutic transference prior to and after psychotherapy. As mentioned earlier, hypnosis was used successfully to desexualize feelings towards males and sexualize feelings toward females. This supports the conclusion that hypnotic influence can, if properly applied, be utilized to favorably alter, rather than to intensify, neurotic transference. By means of hypnoanalysis, resistances can often be promptly and effectively explored, ventilated and resolved in both the hypnotic and posthypnotic state. Efforts were made to potentiate a healthy father-son transference in therapy and normal role identification in terms of masculine behavior toward the opposite sex. In instances, where there is an unconscious desire for homosexual union with the father, hypnotic suggestion can be employed to help desexualize this urge and to encourage an identification with healthy males.

Recently, I treated a 30-year old bisexual who had been seduced by a clever vice squad detective to the point of my patient's sitting down on a park bench next to him, feeling his thigh, whereupon the detective flashed his badge. C. was referred to me by his attorney. His wife was dismayed, shocked and dumbfounded. She hadn't known that C. led a double life.

An initial history was obtained in which C. revealed that he had been reared by a harsh, tyrannical, unloving father and an unhappy, overworked, oppressed mother. Hypnoaversion therapy was instituted. An attempt was made to create an aversion in C. to the smell of males and in particular to the fantasied, horrible breath of males whom he encountered in hypnotically induced fantasies. C. became so averse that he would become intensely nauseous as soon as he was close to a homosexual male. After the sickening experience, hypnotic fantasies were induced to the effect that he ran away from the disgusting situation to a beautiful flower garden where his wife, B. was sitting on a bench. As he moved close to her, it was suggested that he detected her lovely fragrance, and then as he touched, caressed and embraced her, he felt the beautiful softness and warmth and receptiveness of her body. He kissed her passionately in the hypnotic fantasy, clinging to a large soft pillow symbolizing B.

A month after the treatment was initiated twice weekly, C. had completely lost any desire for contact with males. His marital life has become most gratifying and he now engages in sex five to seven times weekly. Adjunctive group and individual psychotherapy was given and C. has developed a warm father transference with the therapist. After seven months of weekly follow-up, C. manifests a very strong sexual love feeling for his wife and has had no reoccurrence of homosexual impulses. Again I wish to emphasize that it is of paramount importance in the treatment to replace the homosexual love object by a gratifying heterosexual one.

Hypnoanalysis was also used to uncover blocked recollections regarding early emotional and sexual development. Furthermore, specific anxieties regarding masculine, aggressive behavior with females were explored under hypnosis and the resultant findings consciously ventilated and discussed. I have found that frequently these anxieties can be markedly lessened and the patient motivated to express more gratifying masculine behavior.

As noted earlier, attempts were made under hypnosis to uncover any specific disgust reactions which patients had experienced during homosexual contact and to potentiate these, with strong suggestion that these would recur on contact with a male body.

In the patients observed, disgust aversion reactions to the male body persevered for months after receiving four to six initial treatments. It is, of course, very advisable to prolong individual treatment and sometimes intensify it until the desired clinical results are well established. The intensity and duration of disgust reactions vary individually, depending to a considerable extent on suggestibility and the degrees of the original disgust reactions.

As an optimum procedure, after the initial treatment period of several months, periodic reinforcement at two to four week intervals is advisable for about one year or longer depending on the patient's response.

The initial clinical results are encouraging and further study of these and additional cases is considered advisable. As indicated earlier, this hypnoaversion procedure also appears to be particularly promising as an adjunctive in the treatment of female homosexuality. It is most important to simultaneously involve the patient in group therapy in a male-female group. (Individual sessions can be held in addition, when indicated.) Involvement in the group therapy offers an excellent opportunity for evaluating the patient's progress and interaction with the opposite sex.

HYPNOAVERSION TREATMENT OF NARCOTICS ADDICTION

Preliminary investigation has provided support of the possibility that hypnoaversion therapy can be of value in the treatment of certain drug addicts. I have experimentally attempted to create an aversion to the needle and to the effects of narcotic drugs in six patients thus far with some success. Recently, I treated a scientist, age 51, who had become addicted to Talwin which he administered by intravenous injection. He related that he could remember one occasion of particular discomfort—feeling of precordial pressure in his chest and marked weakness which upset him immediately following an injection. The injections of a narcotic solution in this case, a Talwin placebo, were simulated and a suggestion given that he would immediately feel the same discomfort in his chest and a feeling of marked weakness. This reaction promptly occurred. The treatment was repeated on successive days for five days, whereupon the patient developed a very marked aversion to the needle and a dread of the effects of the drug. Of interest was the fact that already following the first treatment he had a dream in which he said some male monster was trying to overpower him and inject him with a poisonous drug. This was taken as an obvious good prognostic indication of the effect of treatment. Since the patient lived a distance away, he was taught self-hypnosis so that he could continue to reinforce the effects of the treatment.

Chapter 10

CONTRAINDICATIONS, LIMITATIONS AND ERRORS IN HYPNOTHERAPY

It is highly important that we carefully evaluate the contraindications as well as indications for hypnosis and hypnotherapy. We must be careful to differentiate organic from psychogenic and functional illnesses. There are organic conditions that can derive therapeutic benefits from hypnotherapy, and often a combination of the former with medical treatment can be most advantageous. In this connection, particularly, are conditions such as peptic-duodenal ulcer, diabetes, asthma, hypertension, tachycardia, mucous colitis, and many others. Hypnosis can often be invaluable in differential diagnosis. There are instances in which conditions such as multiple sclerosis have been diagnosed as hysteria and treatment attempted by hypnosis, although the reverse is also true. Just recently, I saw a patient suffering from hysteria who had been treated for three years for multiple sclerosis.

We should not permit the use of hypnosis to satisfy

childish curiosity or fads. There should be a serious and justifiable reason for its application. In most instances, unless there is earnest motivation on the part of the patient for help, treatment is generally of little or no value. In the event there is a resistance to treatment, every effort should be made to first resolve it.

Furthermore, patients should under no circumstances be compelled or strongly influenced to submit to hypnosis. It is much better not to abruptly hypnotize patients but rather to carefully explore their case histories with an attempt to determine their principal problems and needs. A preliminary warm-up and establishment of good rapport is usually most helpful. An attempt should be made to determine to what extent the patient at the particular time is able to face his real problems. Premature presentation and interpretation of deeper conflicts have often resulted in producing disturbing reactions in patients such as marked anxiety, guilt, etc., as well as increasing resistance to treatment. A good background history makes it easier to explore the patient's problems under hypnosis and provides important points of reference.

I heartily concur with Erickson and Wolberg that meaningful motivation plays an important part in the success of hypnotherapy. Further, that the best interests and desires of the patient should be respectfully considered. Such an attitude on the part of the hypnotherapist yields far better results. The therapist in this instance wisely attempts to ally himself with the patient in his pursuit of a satisfactory solution of his problems, thus practically eliminating resistance. The principal aim of therapy should always be the happiness and well-being of the patient. We must seek to relieve the patient of pain and suffering rather than to create it. We must alleviate and, when possible, remove symptoms rather than aggravate and create additional symptoms. Every effort must be made to further the emotional maturity of the patient, to lessen his dependency on the therapy, and to prepare him for the needs of a real world.

COMMON ERRORS

As aforementioned, the patient under hypnosis is very vulnerable and often highly perceptive. Offhand remarks made in the presence of the hypnotized subject to a nurse or colleague can have a marked effect. This type of "eavesdropping" by the patient can be very effectively utilized therapeutically. However, if great care is not exercised, the patient may be deeply traumatized by seemingly innocuous remarks. The therapist must remember that in the hypnotic trance, the patient is highly affective and very vulnerable to suggestion. Even more so, he is literally defenseless against remarks picked up by "eavesdropping." One must remember that the patient under hypnosis is in a relative state of dissociation such that logical thinking and discriminatory functions are reduced. Often remarks directed at someone else may be reacted to as though they were directed at the patient. (Similar to ideas of reference observed in psychosis.)

Many therapists are not fully aware of the impact of their voice and manner on the subject. The hypnotized patient seeks warmth, protection and kindliness from the therapist. A gruff, impatient or irritable voice might disturb the patient markedly. The voice must always be kind, gentle, when necessary, unwavering, strong and sympathetic. I have found in my experience at our clinic that the reactions of the patient are often totally different, depending in large measure on the quality of the voice and manner with which the hypnotist handles the patient. One must not forget to be interested in and sympathetic to the wishes, desires and ultimate ambitions of the patient. The hypnotist must never make the mistake of attempting to dominate the patient, but must rather make him feel that he is helping him to attain his goal. The voice of the hypnotist must also convey sympathy and respect toward the patient. This point of making the patient feel that he is respected and looked up to rather than looked down upon is highly important both from the therapeutic and the rapport viewpoint. The patient often inwardly longs for a feeling of acceptance by the therapist. This is especially significant since the hypnotist assumes an image of importance and authority to the patient. This attitude of unqualified acceptance is particularly important towards patients suffering from feelings of inadequacy, insecurity, and rejection, and in patients who are starved for lack of love. Certainly the utmost consideration should be shown an emotionally disturbed patient in the best interests of a constructive therapeutic approach. This is also very important with patients under hypnosis due to their aforementioned greatly increased affectivity.

Great care must be taken in giving posthypnotic suggestions. It is all too easy to unwittingly create certain compulsions or phobias in the patient and to later have great difficulty in eradicating these. If positive optimistic anticipations are to be planted in the subject's mind, it is important to be certain *a priori* that these can be fulfilled in reality, lest the patient wind up even more disillusioned, despairing and depressed than before. With an improper initial approach, feelings of disillusionment and insecurity may rapidly develop in the patient, since the hypnotist is generally regarded as a sort of omniscient, omnipotent father. However, this idol can rapidly crumble if he fails his patients.

The effect of suggestion greatly depends on the degree of authority which the therapist commands, as well as on rapport. The therapist must always speak with assurance, strength and warmth. One inexperienced hypnotist inadvertently remarked to a patient about to be induced, "Well, I shall try to relax you," whereupon the patient exclaimed, "What do you mean 'try'—I was told that you could!" Colleagues, if you're scared, for heaven's sake, don't let your patient know it.

ERRORS IN TECHNIQUE

In some instances, in spite of the most skillful application of induction technique, the patient may resist relinquishing consciousness. After initial fruitless effort, the hypnotist may inquire into the patient's resistance and discover that the patient was very much concerned with being on time to an important appointment or about her children coming home from school at 3:30—"I was worried whether you'd awaken me in time." On occasion, the patient may resist induction and it is later found that she was concerned about having left her purse containing some valuables in the waiting room. Initial anxieties should be discussed and resolved prior to any induction attempt.

A case in point is that of a patient, from out-of-town, who had been brought in by her family against her will and who revealed marked anxiety. The interview was terminated without an attempt to induce hypnosis. When she was at the door, she remarked, "But I came to get the treatment," to which was replied, "If you wish—I'll be very happy to do so." She then readily submitted to hypnosis. This patient later clearly revealed that she was possessed by a deeper inner conflict between feminine dependency and masculine independency and unconsciously strove to control, dominate and retain the initiative; she felt secure only in a dominant masculine role. She could only cooperate when she made the decision.

As Wolberg and Erickson have repeatedly emphasized, it is therapeutically unwise and unethical to use hypnosis to compel patients to do things which are against their own interests or would in any way impede their treatment. Furthermore, it is simply poor technique to turn the patient against the hypnotist when he can be turned into an ally, a positive asset, thus greatly furthering rapport, transference, cooperation, etc. Patients cooperate best when they feel the hypnotist is entirely in accord with and allied with the realization of their objectives. Patients prior to hypnosis are usually wary and on guard against being abused. Hence, it is highly important to gain their trust. Generally, they will cooperate with the hypnotist to the degree that they have faith and respect for his professional integrity and desire to help them. Experimentally it has been definitely established that they will become disturbed and resistive and generally refuse to carry out asocial acts or to take steps which might compromise them or threaten their security or principles.

The use of hypnosis by parlor playboys, entertainers, magicians and quacks should be strongly discouraged. No one should be permitted to use hypnosis to treat emotional illness unless he has been adequately and properly trained in psychodynamics and has had clinical training under competent professional supervision. Certainly physicians trained in the application of hypnosis to specific medical and surgical problems should be encouraged to use hypnotic techniques. The value of adequate theoretical and clinical training should be stressed. Laws should be established to protect the public from quacks and charlatans who use hypnosis to abuse and take advantage of patients. Such individuals, in the past, have done much to discredit hypnosis as a method of healing. Proper standards of training and ethics should be established. It must be kept in mind that hypnosis is a potent instrument which can not only relieve symptoms but create them. For instance, conditions such as posthypnotic nausea, dizziness and headaches have been reported by some workers. Wolberg has reported observations of spontaneous trances occurring. Such reactions may also occur in hysterical and schizophrenic patients. Erickson has pointed out that such claims as permanent alteration of personality, distortion and falsifications of reality, induction or escape mechanisms, compulsive reactions to immoral suggestions and hypersuggestability resulting from the continued use of hypnosis, although possible, are very much exaggerated.

As for the development of dependency states, this depends upon how the patient is influenced. The patient can be, as a result of hypnotic suggestions, pushed in the direction of greater independence rather than dependence upon the therapist. The therapist must be careful to apply ego-building and strengthening devices so that the patient will take greater independent initiative. Wolberg points out that "whether or not the patient will become dependent seems to reside in his needs rather than in the techniques used." He goes on to add that people having a need for a dependency relationship will become dependent upon the therapist even if he uses a nondestructive passive approach exclusively. Generally, I attempt by hypnosis to strongly encourage and influence a patient to take the initiative in such a manner that he will achieve real successes. As a result of these initial successes, the patient gains ego strength and more initiative and drive. A beneficient cycle is thus set in motion. Important secondary gains can thus often be achieved.

There are, as aforementioned, situational types of resistance, such as, "I have an appointment and I'm afraid I will be late," or "I can't stand anyone looking at me when I am trying to relax." In the latter instance, I have sometimes utilized autohypnosis and permitted the patient to relax while alone. Generally a discussion of the reasons underlying resistance is very beneficial since thereby often basic problems of the patient can be worked through successfully. Attempting to overpower the patient's resistance is definitely unwise. The patient must be permitted the opportunity to work through and resolve his anxieties.

When a patient fails to enter the hypnotic state, a most frequent cause is underlying repressed fear. I recently was treating a 55-year old widow for obesity by hypnoaversion. On the initial induction attempt, she failed to surrender motor control. If, for example, I dropped her arm, she would move it to another position.

When questioned as to whether she had any anxiety about the hypnotic relaxation, she denied such. However, when queried about any incidents she might have had involving a loss of control and consciousness, she recalled that she had had several fainting spells and on one occasion injured herself. Since then, she admitted that she had had a fear of losing consciousness and that this had made it more difficult to fall asleep on occasion. When it was made clear to her that in the hypnotic state one is not unconscious, but that it is merely an altered state of consciousness, that under hypnosis one is not helpless and able to communicate, her fear rapidly dissipated. She was then hypnotized without any difficulty with excellent therapeutic results.

Care should be taken to query the patient on whether he has any hearing deficiency. Sometimes patients explain after failing the initial induction test that they had been unable to hear the hypnotist.

During the hypnotic interview, it is best not to press the interview too rapidly. If this is done, it may produce more anxiety, and anger, and result in blocking resistance on the part of the patient. Longer pauses on the part of the patient in answering are often very meaningful. Material charged with conflict is often given with hesitation, and it is often wise to explore the reasons for such pauses, i.e., the underlying anxiety, resentment, or guilt. The therapist should not reveal disapproval but rather with a kindly, soft and sympathetic tone encourage the patient into further revelation of repressed material. It is often beneficial to give posthypnotic suggestion during the trance so that the patient shall be able to explain his hesitation or manifest resistance consciously upon awakening from the trance.

It is best to explain to patients that hypnosis is not a form of magic which can miraculously cure them. It is wise to point out that hypnosis is a scientific method of healing which can help a patient to communicate and understand his own problems better, that all human problems have specific causes, and that hypnosis is a valuable tool in helping to uncover these causes. One might first point out that hypnosis, like other forms of medical treatment, can be an important adjunct in helping the patient to help himself towards happiness and health, and that his full cooperation is an important factor toward achieving these ends.

Many patients are disturbed by the word "hypnosis." We may generally substitute the term "relaxation." With the endogenic method, the patient is told that he will be relaxed by a psychophysiological method which causes both physical and mental relaxation. In many instances, indirect approaches are better in the induction of the anxious or resistive patients. For instance, the doctor can explain that he wishes to test the patient's ability to relax. This has an added advantage of importance. If the patient fails the test, it is not the doctor who has failed. Thus, the patient will not consider the doctor as incompetent and lose faith. The therapist can encourage the patient at this point by pointing out that with a little helpful discussion, the patient could be tested again and would very likely pass the test. This latter approach worked beautifully recently with a highly suspicious borderline paranoid patient, although he was markedly resistive to the direct approach. Often narcissistic patients are responsive to having their "ability to relax" or any other ability, tested. On one occasion, in a demonstration to a group of doctors, the patient, quite disturbed, stated that she could not possibly relax with the eyes of the doctors upon her. Whereupon she was given instructions on how to relax and all left the room, complying with her wish; she then promptly relaxed into a hypnotic trance. When an induction is attempted in front of a group of professionals, it is best to use the author's auxiliary hypnotist technique. Observers in the group can heighten suggestive influence by confirming the observations of the hypnotist. (See section on auxiliary hypnotist.) Often it is important for the doctor not to press induction too forcefully, but to treat the occasion casually as though there were no pressing indication for using it. Here the "I'll help you if you wish to try" approach is suggested. In resistive or anxious patients, the approach should never be direct. Warming up sessions to promote rapport are often advisable. Another approach, often quite effective, is, "Would you like me to show you how you can relax yourself when you feel nervous or uncomfortable or can't rest?" Many patients resist the idea of an external influence but do not feel similarly about inducing relaxation by themselves. Again, the "I'll help you if you wish to try" approach is suggested. When patients present resistance because they are frightened or disturbed by the idea of being overpowered by an authoritative person, they were countered with the explanation that this was not the purpose of the therapist, that he merely desired to demonstrate how they might learn to relax themselves. Emphasis on the voluntary cooperation of the patient has the further advantage that should the patient resist, the hypnotist can always transfer the responsibility for failure and stress the question as to why the patient couldn't cooperate, etc. In such instances, particularly in the initial attempt, the hypnotist should remain somewhat passively sympathetic and patient. Since many patients are willing to accept only a light state of hypnotic relaxation during the first induction, it is unwise to attempt to push the patient into deeper hypnosis. They are feeling their way and are often unwilling to surrender their conscious selves entirely. It is best to let such patients relax progressively. After several inductions, such patients can often be hypnotized deeply and with great rapidity. During each trance, they should be given posthypnotic suggestion that they will always relax deeper into a trance the next time they go under.

As indicated earlier, under hypnosis there is a state of generally increased hyperaffectivity and hypersensitivity. The patient in the trance is in a highly vulnerable state and can be subject to considerable anxiety, guilt, and emotional disturbance. Thus consideration of the patient's feelings and wishes must be carefully taken into account. Great care must be exercised not to unduly disturb patients in this state, and to avoid creating conflicts and symptoms which may later be difficult to eradicate.

Often patients manifest marked resistance when they are not yet ready to accept interpretations and to relinquish neurotic defenses. They may stubbornly resist change in their personalities. Such attempts may precipitate severe anxiety. The therapist should not be overly energetic in such instances, and first try to mobilize insight, awareness, and understanding as a prelude to accepting the conclusions arrived at.

It is always best *a priori* to discuss the reasons why patients are seeking hypnotherapy and not to offer or propose such treatment indiscriminately. Through such discussions, many erroneous assumptions concerning magical, miraculous and easy cures can be resolved, with the resultant avoidance of damaging disappointment and disillusionment. In some cases that are not responding favorably to conventional therapy, hypnosis can be of great value in furthering communication, recollection and transference. However, it is erroneous to assume that a patient's personality problems will be successfully resolved by means of hypnosis alone. Hypnosis can help to speed up the therapeutic process, but the real and lasting therapeutic benefit comes principally through a conscious working through process and healing transference relationship between patient and therapist or the patient relating to others in a group therapy setting. As noted earlier, material obtained in the hypnotic state should be ventilated and discussed with the patient in the conscious state.

Hypnosis can often help to rapidly explore what the ungratified inner needs of the patient are, thus making it possible to better plan a therapeutic strategy. The adjunctive use of hypnosis can be illustrated in the following example of a middle-aged male patient suffering from severe depression and deep-seated guilt feelings. He was very uncommunicative and avoided social contacts because of these feelings. By means of posthypnotic suggestion, it was possible to bring him into a positive group relationship and group therapy where he felt accepted and was able to communicate with a progressively lesser degree of anxiety. This approach led to a rapid improvement in the patient's condition.

EXCESSIVE DEMANDS

Do not make excessive demands on the hypnotized patient. This can often have very harmful results. In this connection, posthypnotic suggestions were given to a confirmed homosexual patient with whom excellent rapport had been established to the effect that he would henceforth have normal feelings about women, about having a family, children, etc., and that he would feel an aversion to homosexuals. The patient developed a severe headache not long after awakening (symptomatic in this case of acute inner conflict). He became disturbed and restless, and somewhat agitated; began drinking and, after some confused behavior, was arrested in a public toilet for being drunk and disorderly. Later the patient confided that he had desire but was unable to meet the demands made on him at that time, and that these demands had frightened him.

Try to be certain then, that the patient is ready to accept the demands made upon him. Excessive demands often precipitate anxiety, resentment, guilt, and resistance to hypnosis and treatment. A posthypnotic suggestion was given to an aggressively masculine woman that she would be more responsive and passively receptive to her husband in their sexual life. The patient came into such a degree of inner conflict that she abstained from sex altogether, complaining of malaise. Soon after, she was somewhat resistant to hypnotic induction, and when queried consciously about how she felt, she declared in an angry voice, "Doctor, I resent being forced into passive submission to my husband. That's what they always did at home—made me give in father, to brother—to those damned men! If I do it, I want to do it because I feel differently about my role as a woman." Tactics then were changed. Since she experienced no orgasm during coitus, hypnotic suggestion was used to the effect that the more aggressive she was sexually, the greater difficulty she would have attaining gratification; rather, that full sexual gratification could only be achieved through complete feminine acceptance and receptiveness to her husband. She began to unconsciously, progressively associate receptiveness, submission and responsiveness with achieving gratification and the ultimate pleasure of orgasm, and was as a result enabled to have gratifying sex. Her husband was helped to assume a more assertive and actively demonstrative role.

Chapter 11

THE FUTURE OF HYPNOTHERAPY

Hypnosis in medicine has finally found virtually universal acceptance as a healing art. The use of hypnosis in obstetrics has become widespread. As a result not only painless natural childbirth is possible, but with fewer complications such as excessive bleeding or stillbirths. More and more physicians are using hypnosis to advantage. It provides a safe, innocuous method of relieving anxiety, pain and tensions.

More and more psychiatrists and psychologists are studying hypnosis and hypnotherapy. What sense is there in treating conditions such as phobias for months and years by conventional psychotherapy when they can be cleared up in several sessions of hypnotherapy—sometimes in even a single session. Such phobias include height and flying phobia, nyctophobia, assault phobia, injury phobia, and other anxiety states.

When we think in terms of psychotherapy for the many as well as for the few, as my late dear friend, W. Eliasberg put it, we must consider treatment procedures which are not laborious, costly and time-consuming, but rather ones more effective and practical.

Due to the fact that methods of induction have been improved, made more systematic and feasible, hypnosis has become a more effective tool when applied to specific clinical problems. By speeding up hypnotic induction, as for example, with the endogenic method, the use of hypnosis becomes more practical for the busy practitioner. In recent years, much clinical information on the application of hypnosis and hypnotherapy to medicine, surgery, psychotherapy and other areas has been accumulated. The prolongation procedure which I have introduced makes use of hypnoanalgesia and anaesthesia more efficacious for certain surgical procedures.

No doubt, not every one can become a good hypnotist. Not everyone can become a good surgeon, lawyer or engineer. Certainly personality and motivation are factors in one's becoming successful as a hypnotherapist. Most therapists can attain a high level of effectiveness with proper training and supervised practice. Undoubtedly, now that the psychoanalytic bias against the use of hypnotherapy has subsided somewhat and psychotherapists are looking for more practical, rapid and effective techniques, hypnotherapy will be utilized increasingly in psychotherapy, often in conjunction with other approaches.

It is evident that nondirective, passive types of therapists will not function well as hypnotists until they have been able to modify their approach vis-a-vis the patient and become more active and directive. Some can adjust in time and become good hypnotists. Sometimes, the nondirective therapist needs to be convinced that more active therapeutic approaches and specifically hypnosis can yield good results.

Hypnoaversion therapy, which I introduced in 1959 first as an adjunctive treatment for alcoholics, has proven to be highly efficacious in nicotinism, obesity and weight control. As referred to previously, I have employed hypnoaversion therapy in conjunction with hypnoanalysis quite successfully in the treatment of homosexuals of the bisexual type in both males and females.

The great value of hypnosis in differential diagnosis, i.e., distinguishing functional from organic illness, malingering from actual illness, cannot be too strongly emphasized. Take, for example, the case of the 55-year old woman who complained of inability to swallow. (See Chapter seven.)

Hypnosis can be used with surprising benefit in dermatologic disorders, i.e., Darrier's neurodermatoses, urticarias, certain types of eczemas, herpes zoster and lichen ruber planus, in particular, when there are inflammatory-type lesions. Hypnotic suggestion is beneficial in thrombophlebitis, reducing pain and swelling. Because of its antiphilogistic effect, hypnotic suggestion may be beneficial in reducing noninfectious irritative inflammatory lesions generally.

The value of hypnosis in obstetrics is considerable. It is of use not only in making painless natural birth without drugs possible, in reducing the number of stillbirths, in facilitating labor, in reducing bleeding, but it can be very useful in pre-and postnatal care. Patients can be instructed and trained to follow the correct treatment regime.

A high percentage of gynecological disorders are of functional etiology, i.e., conditions such as pseudocyesis, functional ammenorrhea, dysmenorrhea, vaginismus, frigidity and many others, may respond well to hypnotherapy if properly employed.

The value of hypnosis in dentistry has been amply demonstrated, i.e., relieving anxiety, discomfort and pain. It can be used in orthodontic work, in teeth repair, in prosthetics, fillings, and in some instances, even in extractions, particularly if there is a sensitivity to the use of novocaine and adrenaline. Certainly preoperative use of hypnotic suggestion can greatly reduce emotional trauma. Hypnosis is also useful in relaxing patients and relieving tension and pain when probing sensitive teeth. Hypnotic relaxation and suggestion can be quite helpful in helping patients become better adjusted to wearing dental plates for the first time.

Hypnotherapy is of unquestionable benefit in certain cases of asthma. I have found hypnosis to be effective in bronchial relaxation, due to relaxation of smooth muscle. Furthermore, as indicated earlier, it can be of marked value in the aborting of migraine attacks. Moreover hypnosis may be used successfully to explore the emotional causes of asthma or migraine attacks. Hypnotherapy can be invaluable in the treatment of sexual problems, i.e., impotence, frigidity, perversion and aversion.

Hypnosis, I have found, can be used very effectively to markedly potentiate the effects of certain drugs, i.e., testosterone, estrogens, and placebos, as well. Hypnosis has proven to be of increasing value in police and legal work, in particular, in obtaining evidence. Hypnosis because it facilitates memory can sometimes aid witnesses in recalling details surrounding a crime. It appears that in the hypnotic state affectivity is increased. It is my view that specific feelings trigger off intellectual recall and repressed traumatic memories. Narcohypnosis and hypnosis may be important in determining motives for crimes and details surrounding the commitment of the offense.

If hypnotherapy can be highly effective in the treatment of phobias and fears of injury, it may also be of value in the treatment of compulsive-obsessive disorders which are often so resistive to therapy. In compulsive-obsessive patients there are deeply repressed fears. One might call compulsive behavior an unconscious defense against fear, an attempt to ward off the dreaded danger. There is definite evidence that hypnotherapy can be very valuable in the treatment of depressive conditions, particularly in diverting rage away from the self, relieving guilt, despair, venting hurts, emphasizing positive suggestions, i.e., joyous, healthy recreation, etc.

Hypnosis can be of considerable value in rehabilitation work. Persons with limb impairment needing motivation to continue active exercises and retraining for the use of artificial limbs and new muscles can benefit greatly from posthypnotic suggestions. Such hypnotic conditioning can be of great value in many psychomotor activities, i.e., typing, computer training, sewing, operating vehicles, etc.

I have found hypnosis to be of great value in helping performers, lecturers, teachers and executives in overcoming fears of facing audiences and speaking effectively. Likewise, it can be of great help in stage and performance fright.

I was on one occasion consulted by a scientist, who was in an executive position with a large corporation. He was very troubled by his marked apprehension in facing audiences and presenting scientific material. He had seen me only once due to the pressure of business matters. Then six weeks later I received a surprise telephone call from the West Coast. On the telephone he was extremely apprehensive about having to face an audience of industrialists and scientific experts in a presentation he had been assigned to make for his company. "I have to give this presentation in one hour, and I can't face it," he exclaimed. My answer was that if he had to make the presentation in an hour further discussion would be useless and that I would immediately hypnotize him. This I proceeded to do via the telephone and gave suggestions to the effect that he would feel very confident because he had such an excellent grasp of the material, and that he would give a fine presentation. After offering the suggestions, he was brought out of the trance. I later learned that he gave an excellent presentation and was very gratified with the result.

Hypnotherapy is a relatively new field as far as its broad application is concerned. With the great increase in the use of hypnosis in medicine and psychiatry and a stepping up of clinical research in hypnosis, new applications and more effective methods will undoubtedly be developed.

Hypnotherapy, without a doubt, has a great future and increasingly progressive and farsighted therapists will make use of this important clinical tool. It is obviously senseless to undergo months and years of psychoanalytic treatment for relief of a condition that could be readily resolved in several hypnotherapeutic sessions. Often the therapeutic results are rapid and encouraging to the patient. Certainly in deep-seated conditions, the period of therapy can be shortened by the use of hypnosis to explore causative factors and motivate the patient therapeutically.

Hypnotherapy can be of particular value in crisis intervention. In such situations procrastination and delay may have serious consequences. There are situations in which rapid effective release of tensions and violently destructive feelings can be decisive in the prevention of tragic consequences. It can be a rapid, effective tool in forestalling serious complications and tragedies. For example, I have employed hypnocatharsis very successfully in forestalling homicidal and suicidal acts. In fact, such acts can be enacted in fantasy with the usual remorse, guilt and fears experienced as an aftermath, thus forestalling the actual commitment of the violent acts. Under hypnosis, it is possible to rapidly release pent-up rage directed at others or at oneself. Furthermore, under hypnosis, the sources of such rage can be promptly explored. It was possible in a number of cases to give post hypnotic suggestions so that the violent act was acted out on the stage instead of in reality. This procedure is now to be employed at our projected suicide-homicide prevention center in South Jersey. The need for methods for rapid intervention in critical situations is obvious.

As I have stated earlier, hypnotherapy has been yielding splendid results in the treatment of nicotinism. It has been possible to cure the smoking addiction in many cardiovascular and respiratory diseased patients who were unable to stop smoking without help.

Hypnotherapy can be of great value in the treatment of speech problems, such as stammering, stuttering, etc. as well as in speech retraining. It can be of most value in uncovering the underlying neurotic speech defense mechanisms and the causes relating back to childhood.

Hypnotherapy can be of great value in helping persons to overcome learning blocks, i.e., especially in learning languages, reading, or learning how to study. Of interest is the case of a 23-year old female graduate student who was in an acute depression because the dean of the college had notified her that she was about to fail out of the program. My patient became extremely depressed and suicidal. She felt there was no future, no hope for her now that she was being dropped from graduate school. She felt very guilty toward her mother, a retired school teacher and widow living on a small pension. She had supported her through college and how could she face her mother now? After a strenuous appeal, the dean allowed my patient to remain, pending the outcome of treatment. Intensive hypnotherapy was started. Another graduate student, a former patient of mine, who had graduated with honors in the same department, prepared the study plan for the patient. The material was fed in by suggestion, while hypnosis was utilized to motivate not only studying but the faithful carrying out of all her academic obligations. To make a long story short, after a period of five months of hypnotherapy, the patient graduated cum laude.

Hypnotic suggestion can be of great help in behavior modification and habit training. It can be very useful in rehabilitation, i.e., training a person to use the left hand in place of an incapacitated or absent right hand, or to learn how to walk on artificial limbs, etc.

To review, in summary, some of the principal clinical

applications of therapeutic hypnosis are in connection with its use in the following areas:

1. Differential diagnosis
2. Uncovering repressed material (hypnoanalysis)
3. Behavioral modification
4. Symptom alleviation, removal or displacement
5. Treatment of phobias (sexual and social anxiety, hypnodesensitization)
6. Motivational stimulation
   a. Toward social participation
   b. To increase cooperation in the treatment program, i.e., adhering to dietary and/or exercise regimes, etc.
   c. To aid patients who are suffering physical disabilities, to exercise limbs, etc.
   d. To increase personal effectiveness in study or work situations
7. To relieve pain
   a. Headaches
   b. In particular, all forms of psychogenic pain
   c. In anaesthesia
      1. Obstetrics
      2. Dentisty
      3. Minor surgery
8. To alleviate anxiety
   a. Preoperative anxiety
   b. Interpersonal anxiety (overcoming anxiety, e.g., related to participating and communicating in groups)
   c. School or work anxieties

I should like at this point to caution against the consideration of hypnosis and hypnotherapy as a panacea. Clinical experience has clearly demonstrated to me that no single system of psychotherapy is complete and adequate for treating every problem. Hypnosis is, after all, another method of communicating with patients. It can be, if properly employed, of great diagnostic and therapeutic value. There are so many conditions in which hypnotic techniques have proven to be of marked and often decisive importance. We are all familiar with the outstanding therapeutic results of such hypnotherapists as Erickson, Van Pelt, Wolberg, Kline, Salter, Rosen, and others.

The author's method of endogenic hypnosis is particularly well adapted for teaching patients to prevent or relieve pain or anxiety states by autohypnosis.

I have had several patients who successfully relaxed themselves into hypnosis before undergoing major surgery. They suffered far less psychic trauma and required considerably less anaesthesia. Not the least valuable aspect, of course, is in the field of social psychiatry, where family problems, juvenile delinquency, and addictions are involved.

The future of hypnotherapy depends to a large extent on the ability, ingenuity and training of the new generation of hypnotherapists. Hypnotherapy, in order not to fall into disrepute as a result of poorly trained and incompetent individuals practicing it requires special aptitudes, training and skills.

In recent years, new clinical applications for the use of hypnosis have been developed. When one thinks of how much unnecessary human suffering may be allayed by the use of hypnosis, for example, in stilling the pains of migraine headaches or of terminal cancer patients, and in making possible less painful and safer childbirth, the great promise therapeutic hypnosis holds for the future becomes clear.

REFERENCES

CHAPTER 1—HISTORICAL BACKGROUND OF HYPNOTHERAPY

Baudowin, C., *Suggestion and Autosuggestion,* translated by Eden and Cedar Paul, Allen & Unwin, London, 1920.

Bechterew, W. V., What is hypnosis: *Journal of Abnormal Psychology,* 18–25, 1: April 1906.

Bernheim, H. *Suggestive Therapeutics,* translated by C. A. Herter, Putman's, New York, 1899.

Binet, A. and Fere, C. *Animal Magnetism,* D. Appleton & Co., New York, 1888.

Braid, J., *Neuryphonogy,* George Redway, London, 1899.

Bramwell, J. M., Hypnotism, Wm. Rider & Sons, London, 1913.

Bramwell, J. M., *Hypnotism: Its History, Practice, and Theory,* Lippincott, Philadelphia, (Revised Ed.), 1928.

Breuer, J. and Freud, S., *Studies in Hysteria,* Nervous and Mental Disease Publishing Co., New York, 1936.

Brooks, C. H., *The Practice of Autosuggestion by the Method of Emile Love,* Dodd, Mead, New York, 1922.

Charcot, J. M. *Lectures on the Diseases of the Nervous System,* The New Sydenham Society, London, 1877.

Charcot, J. M. *Oeuvres Completes, Metallotherapie et Hypnotisme,* Bourneville et E. Brissand, Paris, 1890.

Du Bois, Burden, C. and Dubois, F. d'A, *Histoire Academique du Magnetisme Animal: Accompagne's de Notes et de Remarques, Critiques sur Toutes les Observations et Experiences Faites Jusju A Ce Jour, Paris, 1841.*

Elliotson, J., *Numerous Cases of Surgical Operations Without Pain in the Mesmeric State,* London, 1843.

Erickson, M. H. The Applications of Hypnosis to Psychiatry. *Medical Record,* 60–65, July 19, 1939

Erickson, M. H., Hypnotic psychotherapy, The *Medical Clinics of North America,* 32:571–583, 1948.

Esdaile, J., *Natural and Mesmeric Clairvoyance,* Hippolyte Baillière, London, 1852.

Forel, A., *Hypnotism and Psychotherapy,* Translated by H. W. Armit, Rebman, New York, 1907.

Grinker, R. R., Conference on narcosis, hypnosis, and war neuroses, sponsored by the Josiah Macy, Jr. Foundation, New York, January, 1944 (Privately distributed).

Janet, P., *Psychological Healing,* Macmillan, New York, 1925.

Kline, M. V., Freud and hypnosis: a critical evaluation, *British Journal Medical Hypnotism,* 2:1, 1953.

Kroger, W. S., *Clinical and Experimental Hypnosis,* Lippincott, Philadelphia, 1963.

Kubie, L. S. and Margolin, S., *A Physiological Method for the Inductions of Partial Sleep, etc.,* Transactions of the American Neurological Association, 1942.

Liebeault, A., *Du Sommeil et des Etats, Analogues, etc.,* Vienna, Duetricke, 1892.

Lindner, R. M., *Rebel without a Cause, The Hypnoanalysis of a Criminal Psychopath,* Grune & Stratton, Inc., New York, 1944, 289 pages.

McDowell, M., *Hypnosis in Modern Medicine,* Ed. Schneck, Charles C. Thomas, Springfield, Ill., 1953.

Meares, A., *A System of Medical Hypnosis,* Saunders, Philadelphia, 1960.

Mesmer, A., *Memoire sur la Découverte du Magnétisme Animal,* Genéve, 1779.

Mesmer, A., *System Der Wechselwirungen Theorie und Anwendung des Thierischen Magnetisimus als die Allgemeine Heilkunde Zue Erhaltung Des Menschen, Herausgegeben Von Wolfort,* Berlin, 1814.

Moll, A. *Hypnotism,* Translated by A. F. Hopkirk, Charles Scribner's Sons, New York, 1913.

Prince, M., *Clinical and Experimental Studies in Personality,* Ed. A. A. Roback, Sci-Arts, Cambridge, 1939.

Sidis, B. and Goodhart, S. P., *Multiple Personality*, D. Appleton & Co., New York, 1905.

Van Pelt, S. J., Hypnotherapy in medical practice, *British Journal Medical Hypnosis*, 1:8–13, 1949.

Van Pelt, S. J., *Hypnotism and the Power Within*, Baillière, Tindall & Cox, London, 1950.

Van Pelt, S. J., The Control of the heart rate by hypnotic suggestion, in *Experimental Hypnosis*, Ed. Le Cron, The Macmillian Co., New York, 1952.

Wolberg, L., B. *Hypnoanalysis*, Grune & Stratton, New York, 1945.

Yellowlees, H., *A Manual of Psychotherapy*, A & C. Black, London, 1923.

CHAPTER 2—CHARACTERISTICS OF THE HYPNOTIC STATE

Alrutz, S., Die suggestive vesikation, *J. F. Psycholol. U. Neurol.*, 21:1–10, 1915.

Bass, M. J., Differentiation of the hypnotic trance from normal sleep, *Journal of Experimental Psychology*, 14:382–399, 1931.

Benett, T. I. and J. F. Venables, The effect of emotions on the gastric secretion and motility of the human being, *British Medical Journal*, 2:662–663, 1920.

Bernheim, H., *Suggestive Therapeutics*, translated by C. A. Herter, Putnam's, New York, 1899.

Bernheim, H., *Suggestive Therapeutics: a Treatise of the Nature and Uses of Hypnotism*, Translated by C. A. Herter, Putnam's, New York, 1900.

Björstorm, F., *Hypnotism*, translated by Baron Nils, Posse, Humboldt Publishing Co., New York, 1887.

Brenman, M. and Gill, M., *Hypnotherapy*, International Universities Press, New York, 1947.

Breuer, J. and Freud, S., *Studies in Hysteria*, Nervous and Mental Disease Publishing Co., New York, 1936.

Dunlap, K., *Habits, Their Making and Unmaking*, Liveright, New York, 1933.

Estabrooks, E. H., Experimental studies in suggestion, *Journal of Genetic Psychology*, 36:120–139, 1929.

Estabrooks, G. H., *Hypnotism*, Dutton, New York, 1945.

Eysenck, H. S., An experimental study of the improvement of mental and physical functions in the hypnotic state, *British Journal Medical Psychology*, 36:120–139, 1929.

Ferenczi, S., *Further Contributions to the Theory and Technique of Psychoanalysis*, compiled by J. Rickman, translated by J. I. Suttie, Hogarth, London, 1926.

Forel, A., *Hypnotism*, translated by H. W. Armit, Rebman, New York, 1907.

Hart, H. H., Hypnosis in psychiatric clinics, *Journal of Nervous and Mental Diseases*, 74:598–609, 1931.

Heller, F. and Schultz, J. H., Uber einen Fall hypnotisch erzengter Blasenbilding, *Munchen. Med. Wehnschr.*, 56:2112, 1909.

Janet, P., *Principles of Psychotherapy*, Macmillan Co., New York, 1924.

Janet, P. *Psychological Healing*, Macmillan Co., New York, 1925.

Loomis, A. L., Harvey, E. N., and Hobart, G., Brain potentials during hypnosis, *Science*, 83, 239–241, 1936.

Meares, A., *A System of Medical Hypnosis*, Saunders, Philadelphia.

Pavlov, I. P., Inhibition, hypnosis and sleep, *British Medical Journal*, 256–267, 1923a.

Pavlov, I. P., The identity of inhibition with sleep and hypnosis, *Scientific Monthly*, 17, 603–608, 1923b.

Pavlov, I. P., *Conditioned Reflexes: Investigation of Physiological Activities of Cerebral Cortex*, Oxford University Press, London, 1927.

Pavlov, I. P. *Lectures on Conditioned Reflexes*, translated by W. H. Gantt, International Publishers, New York, 1928.

Prince, M. *The Unconscious*, Macmillan Co., New York, 1929.

Salter, A. What is Hypnosis? New York: Richard R. Smith, 1944.

Schilder, P. and Kauders, O., *Hypnosis*, translated by S. Rothenberg, Nervous and Mental Disease Publishing Co., New York, 1927.

Van Pelt, S. J., *Hypnotism and the Power within*, Bailliere, Tindall & Cox, London, 1952.

Wible, C. L. and Jenness, A. Electrocardiograms during sleep and hypnosis, *Journal of Psychology*, 1, 235–245, 1936.

CHAPTER 3—PREPARATION OF THE PATIENT FOR INDUCTION

Braid, J. *Neurypnology; Or, The Rationale of Nervous Sleep, Considered in Relation With Animal Magnetism*. George Redway, London, 1899.

Heyer, G., *Hypnosis and Hypnotherapy*, C. W. Daniel Company, London, 1931.

Lloyd, B. L., *Hypnotism in the Treatment of Disease*, Bale & Danielsson, London, 1934.

Weitzenhoffer, A. M., *General Techniques of Hypnotism,* Grune & Stratton, New York, 1957.

Weitzenhoffer, A. M., *Hypnotism: An Objective Study in Suggestibility,* Chapman & Hall, London, 1953 (Paperbound edition, 1963).

White, M. M., The physical and mental trails of individuals susceptible to hypnosis, *Journal of Abnormal and Social Psychology,* 25:293–298, 1930.

CHAPTER 4—HYPNOTIC INDUCTION

Braid, J., *Neurypnology,* George Redway, London, 1899.

Liebeault, A., *Du Sommeil et des Etats,* Analogues, etc., Vienna, Duetricke, 1892.

Salter, A., Three Techniques of Autohypnosis. Journal of General Psychology, 24:423–438, 1941.

Sargent, W., Camb, M. B., and Fraser, R., Inducing light hypnosis by hyperventilation, *Lancet,* 2:778, 1948.

Schultz, J. H. and Luthe, W., *Autogenic Training,* Grune & Stratton, New York, 1959.

CHAPTER 5—MANIFESTATIONS AND HANDLING OF RESISTANCE TO HYPNOTIC INDUCTION

Erickson, M. H. The use of automatic drawing in the interpretation and relief of a state of acute obsessional depression, *Psychoanalytic Quarterly,* 7:443–466, 1938.

Erickson, M. H. and Hill, L., Unconscious mental activity in hypnosis, psychoanalytic implications, *Psychoanalytic Quarterly,* 13:60–78, 1944.

Meares, A., *A System of Medical Hypnosis,* Saunders, Philadelphia, 1960.

Miller, M. M., New and simpler procedure for hypnotic relaxation and prolongation, Proc. Fourth Int. Conf. Psychotherapy, Barcelona, Sept., 1958.

Watkins, J. C., Antisocial compulsions induced under hypnotic trance, *Journal of Abnormal & Social Psychology,* 42:256, 1947.

Weitzenhoffer, A. M., *Hypnotism,* John Wiley & Sons, Inc., New York, 1953.

Wolberg, L. R., *Hypnoanalysis,* Grune & Stratton, New York, 1945.

CHAPTER 6—CONSIDERATIONS IN CONDUCTING THE HYPNOTIC SESSION

Alrutz, S., Die suggestive vesikation, *J. F. Psychol. U. Neurol.*, 21:1–10, 1915.

Estabrooks, G. H., *Hypnotism*, Dutton, New York, 1945.

Forel, A., *Hypnotism*, translated by H. W. Armit, Rebman, New York, 1907.

Freud, S., *Group Psychology and the Analysis of the Ego*, authorized translation by James Strachey, Hogarth Press, London, 1948.

Heller, F. and Schultz, J. H., Uber einen fall hypnotisch erzeugter blasenbildung, *Munchen. Med. Wehnsche*, 56:2112, 1909.

Loomis, A. L., Harvey, E. N., and Hobart, G., Brain potentials during Hypnosis, *Science*, 83:239–241, 1936.

Schilder, P. and Kauders, O., *Hypnosis*, translated by S. Rothenberg, Nervous and Mental Diseases Publishing Co., New York, 1927.

Schultz, J. H. and Luthe, W., *Autogenic Training*, Grune & Stratton, New York, 1959.

Van Pelt, S. J., *Hypnotism and the Power Within*, Skeffington, London, 1950.

CHAPTER 7—HYPNOTHERAPY AND PSYCHOTHERAPY

Adler, D. L., The experimental production of repression, Proceedings of the 8th Annual Meeting of Topological Psychologists, pp. 27–36, 1940.

Bergler, M. D., *Battle of the Conscience*, Washington Institute of Medicine, Washington, 1948.

Erickson, M. H., Concerning the nature and character of posthypnotic behavior, *Journal of General Psychology*, 24:95–133, 1941a.

Erickson, M. H., The successful treatment of a case of acute hysterical depression by a return under hypnosis to a critical phase of childhood. *Journal of General Psychology*, 24, 95–133, 1941b.

Erickson, M. H., The applications of hypnosis to psychiatry, *Medical Record*, 150:60–65, 1939.

Ferenczi, S., *Theory and Technique of Psychoanalysis*, Boni & Liveright Co., New York, 1927.

Freud, S., *The Psychopathology of Everyday Life*, Macmillan Co., New York, 1914.

Jones, E., The action of suggestion in psychotherapy, *Journal of Abnormal Psychology,* 5:217–254, 1910.

Kanzer, M. G., The therapeutic use of dreams induced by hypnotic suggestion, *Psychoanalytic Quarterly,* 14:313, 1945.

Kroger, W. S., *Clinical and Experimental Hypnosis,* Lippincott, Philadelphia, 1965.

Miller, M. M., Hypnoaversion in the treatment of obesity, *Journal of National Medical Association,* 66:480–481, 1974.

Miller, M. M., Hypnoaversion treatment of nicotinism, *Journal of National Medical Association,* 57:480–482, 1956.

Miller, M. M. *New and Simpler Procedure for Hypnotic Relaxation and Prolongation,* Proc. Fourth Int. Conf. Psychothery., Barcelona, Sept. 1958; Endogenic Hypnosis: Simpler and More Effective Procedure for Hypnotic Induction and Prolongation, Am. J. Social Psychiat. 1:24–30 (Autumn) 1959.

Miller, M. M., Treatment of chronic alcoholism by hypnotic aversion, *Journal of the American Medical Association* 171:1492–1495, 1959.

Miller, M. M., Hypnoaversion treatment in alcoholism, nicotinism and weight control, *Journal of the National Medical Association* 68:129–130, 1976.

Salter, A., *Conditioned Reflex Therapy: The Direct Approach To The Reconstruction of Personality,* Farrar, Straus, and Giroux, Inc. (Capricorn Books Edition) New York, 1949, 1961.

Speyer, N. and Strokvis, B., The psychoanalytic factor in hypnosis, *British Journal of Medical Psychology,* 17:217–222, 1938.

Stekel, W., *Psychoanalysis and Suggestion Therapy,* Kegan Paul, London, 1923.

Taylor, W. S., Behavior under hypnoanalysis and the mechanism of neurosis, *Journal of Abnormal Psychology,* 18:109–124, 1923.

Voegtlin, W. L., Treatment of alcoholism by establishing conditioned reflex, *American Journal of Medicine and Science,* 199:802–810, 1940.

Wolberg, L. R., *Hypnoanalysis,* Grune & Stratton, New York, 1945.

CHAPTER 8—CLINICAL APPLICATIONS OF HYPNOSIS IN VARIOUS SPECIALTIES

Ambrose, G. & Newbold, G., *A handbook of medical hypnosis; an introduction for practitioners and students,* 3d. ed. Baltimore: Williams and Williams Co., 1968.

Bramwell, M., *Hypnotism: Its History, Practice, and Theory*, Lippincott, Philadelphia, 1928 (Revised Ed.), 480 pages.

DeLee, J. B. and Greenhill, J. P., *Principles and Practice of Obstetrics*, W. B. Saunders Co., Philadelphia, 1949.

Deutsch, H., *Psychology of Women*, Vols. I and II, Grune & Stratton, New York, 1944–45.

Dunbar, F., *Emotions and Bodily Changes*, Columbia Univ. Press, New York, p. 335, 1938.

Finer, B. L., Hypnosis as a psychosomatic weapon in the anesthesiologist's armory, in *Hypnosis and Psychosomatic Medicine*, Ed. Lassner, J., Springer-Verlag, New York, pp. 96–99, 142, 1967.

Finer, B. L. and Nylen, B. D., Cardiac arrest in the treatment of burns and report on hypnosis as a substitute for anesthesia, *Plastic Reconstructive Surgery*, 27: 49–55, 142, 1961.

Fisher, C., Hypnosis in treatment of neuroses due to war and to other causes, *War Medicine*, 4:565–76, 1934.

Fisher, V. E. and Morrow, A. J., Experimental Study of Moods, *Character and Personality*, 2:201–208, 1934.

Forel, A., *Hypnotism*, Allied Publications, New York, 1949.

Goldie, L., The medical use of hypnotism, *British Medical Journal*, 2, 1957.

Heilig, R. and Hoff, H., Beitrage zur hypnotischen beeinflussung der magenfunktion, *Med. Klin.*, 21:162–163, 1925a.

Heilig, R. and Hoff, H.: Uber hypnotische beeinflussung der nierenfunktion, *Deutsche Med. Wehnschr.*, 51:1615–1616, 1925b.

Heyer, G. *Hypnosis and Hypnotherapy* London: C. W. Daniel Co., 1931.

Kroger, W. S., and Freed, S. C., *Psychosomatic Gynecology*, Philadelphia, pp. 122–123, 1951.

Miller, M. Proceedings of D.C. Medical Society, Section on Neurology and Psychiatry, Washington, D.C., Sept. 1952.

Newbold, G., *Medical Hypnosis*, Gollancz, London, Ch. 8, 1953.

Read, G. D., *Childbirth Without Fear*, Harper & Brothers, New York, 1944.

Schneck, J. M., *Hypnosis in Modern Medicine*, Charles C. Thomas, Springfield, Ill., 1953.

CHAPTER 9—HYPNOAVERSION THERAPY

Bechterew, W. V., What is hypnosis? *Journal of Abnormal Psychology*, 1:18–25, April, 1906.

Bramwell, J. M., *Hypnotism, Its History, Practice and Theory*, Rider, London, 1930.

Freud, S., *Collected Papers*, Hogarth Press & Institute of Psychoanalysis, London, Vols. I–V.

Marcuse, F. L., *Hypnosis—Fact and Fiction*, Penguin, Harmondsworth, 1959.

Meares, A., *A System of Medical Hypnosis*, Saunders, Philadelphia, 1960.

Miller, M. M., Hypnoaversion treatment in alcoholism, nicotinism and weight control, *Journal of the National Medical Association*, 68:129–130, 1976.

Miller, M. M., Hypnoaversion in the treatment of obesity, *Journal of the National Medical Association*, 66:480–481, 1974.

Miller, M. M., Hypnoaversion treatment of nicotinism, *Journal of the National Medical Association*, 57:480–482, 1956.

Miller, M. M. New and simpler procedure for hypnotic relaxation and prolongation, Proc. Fourth Int. Conf. Psychothery., Barcelona, Sept. 1958; Endogenic Hypnosis: Simpler and more Effective Procedure for Hypnotic Induction and Prolongation, Am. J. Social Psychiat. 1:24–30 (Autumn) 1959.

Miller, M. M., Treatment of chronic alcoholism by hypnotic aversion, *Journal of the American Medical Association*, 171:1492–1495, 1959.

Pavlov, I. P., Inhibition, hypnosis, and sleep, *British Medical Journal*, 256–267, 1923.

Salter, A., Three techniques of autohypnosis, *Journal of General Psychology*, 24:423–438, 1941.

Stekel, W., *The Homosexual Neurosis*, Emerson Books, Inc., New York, 1922.

Voegthn, W. L., Treatment of alcoholism by establishing conditioned reflex, *American Journal of Medicine and Science*, 199:802–810, 1940.

Volgyesi, F. A., *Menschen-Und Tierhypnose*, Zurich, Orell Fussli, (Eng. trans. *Hypnosis in Man and Animals*, Bailliere, Tindall & Cassell, London, 1966.)

CHAPTER 10—CONTRAINDICATIONS, LIMITATIONS AND ERRORS IN HYPNOSIS

Erickson, M. H., Concerning the nature and character of post-hypnotic behavior, *Journal of General Psychology*, 24, 95–133, 1941.

Wolberg, L. R., *Hypnoanalysis*, Grune & Stratton, New York, 1945.

Wolberg, L. R., *Therapy through Hypnosis*, London, Elek, 1953.

CHAPTER 11—THE FUTURE OF HYPNOTHERAPY

Erickson, M. H., The applications of hypnosis to psychiatry, *Medical Record,* 150:60–65, 1939.

Kline, M. V., *Freud and hypnosis: The interaction of psychodynamics and hypnosis.* New York: Julian Press, 1958.

Rosen, H., "The Hypnotic and Hypnotherapeutic Control of Severe Pain," *American Journal of Psychiatry,* 107:917, 1951.

Rosen, H., The hypnotic and hypnotherapeutic unmasking, intesification and recognition of an emotion, *American Journal of Psychiatry,* 109:120, 1952.

Salter, A., Auto hypnosis and habit control, *Therapy through Hypnosis,* Ed. R. H. Rhodes, Citadel Press, New York, pp. 246–248.

Van Pelt, S. J., *Hypnotism and the Power Within,* Skeffington & Son, London, 1952.

Van Pelt, S. J., The control of the heart-rate by hypnotic suggestion, in *Experimental Hypnosis,* (Ed. Le Cron), The Macmillan Co., New York, 1952.

Volgyesi, F. A., *Menschen-und Tierhypnose, ,* Zurich, Urell Fusli, (Eng. trans. *Hypnosis in Man and Animals,* Baillière, Tindall & Cassell, London, 1966.)

Wolberg, L. R., *Hypnoanalysis,* Grune & Stratton, New York, 1945.

INDEX